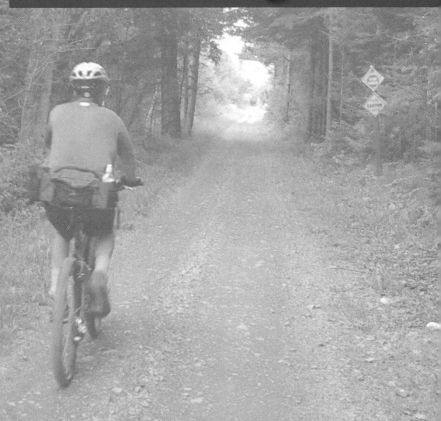

The Official
Rails-to-Trails
Conservancy
Guidebook

D0833427

Rail-Trails
New England

Rail-Trails: New England

1st EDITION June 2007
6th printing 2014

Copyright © 2007 by Rails-to-Trails Conservancy

Front cover photographs copyright © 2007 by Rails-to-Trails
Conservancy
Back cover photograph by Boyd Loving
All interior photographs by Rails-to-Trails Conservancy except for the ones
noted on page 213.

Maps: Gene Olig and Lohnes+Wright

Map data courtesy of: Environmental Systems Research Institute
Cover design: Lisa Pletka and Barbara Richey
Book design and layout: Lisa Pletka
Book editors: Jennifer Kaleba, Karen Stewart, Susan Weaver,
and David Lauterborn

ISBN: 978-0-89997-449-1

Manufactured in the United States of America

Published by: **Wilderness Press**
                  c/o Keen Communications
                  PO Box 43673
                  Birmingham, AL 35243
                  (800) 443-7227; FAX (205) 326-1012
                  info@wildernesspress.com
                  www.wildernesspress.com

Visit our website for a complete listing of our books and for ordering
information.

Distributed by Publishers Group West

Cover photos: Maine's Newport–Dover-Foxcroft
                    Rail-Trail *(main image)*; Connecticut's Housatonic
                    Rail-Trail – Monroe *(upper left)*; New Hampshire's
                    Rockingham Recreational Trail *(lower right)*;
                    Connecticut's Hop River State Park Trail *(back cover)*

Title page photo: Connecticut's Moosup Valley State Park Trail

SAFETY NOTICE: Although Wilderness Press and Rails-to-Trails Conservancy
have made every attempt to ensure that the information in this book is accurate at
press time, they are not responsible for any loss, damage, injury, or inconvenience
that may occur to anyone while using this book. You are responsible for your
own safety and health while in the wilderness. The fact that a trail is described in
this book does not mean that it will be safe for you. Be aware that trail conditions
can change from day to day. Always check local conditions and know your own
limitations. .

About Rails-to-Trails Conservancy

Headquartered in Washington, DC, Rails-to-Trails Conservancy (RTC) fosters one great mission: to protect America's irreplaceable rail corridors by transforming them into multiuse trails. Its hope is that these pathways will reconnect Americans with their neighbors, communities, nature, and proud history.

Railways helped build America. Spanning from coast to coast, these ribbons of steel linked people, communities, and enterprises, spurring commerce and forging a single nation that bridges a continent. But in recent decades, many of these routes have fallen into disuse, severing communal ties that helped bind Americans together.

When RTC opened its doors in 1986, the rail-trail movement was in its infancy. While there were some 250 miles of open rail-trails in the United States, most projects focused on single, linear routes in rural areas, created for recreation and conservation. RTC sought broader protection for the unused corridors, incorporating rural, suburban, and urban routes.

Year after year, RTC's efforts to protect and align public funding with trail building created an environment that allowed trail advocates in communities all across the country to initiate trail projects. These ever-growing ranks of trail professionals, volunteers, and RTC supporters have built momentum for the national rail-trails movement. As the number of supporters multiplied, so too did the rail-trails. By the turn of the 21st century, there were some 1100 rail-trails on the ground, and RTC recorded nearly 84,000 supporters, from business leaders and politicians to environmentalists and healthy-living advocates.

Americans now enjoy more than 13,000 miles of open rail-trails. And as they flock to the trails to commune with neighbors, neighborhoods, and nature, their economic, physical, and environmental wellness continue to flourish.

In 2006, Rails-to-Trails Conservancy celebrated 20 years of creating, protecting, serving, and connecting rail-trails. Boasting more than 100,000 members and supporters, RTC is the nation's leading advocate for trails and greenways.

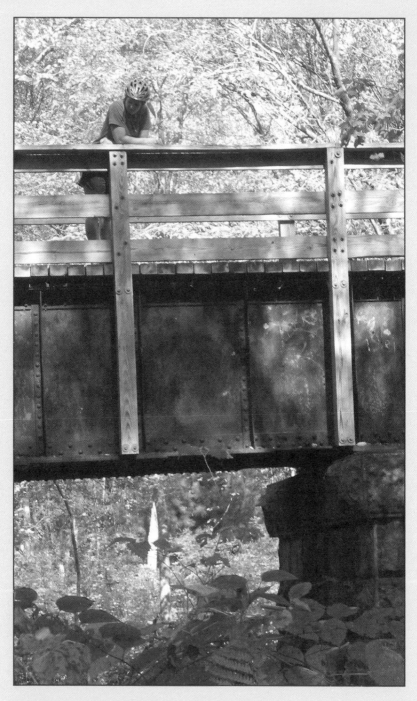

A decked railroad bridge on Connecticut's Moosup Valley State Park Trail

Foreword

Dear Reader:

For those of you who have already experienced the sheer enjoyment and freedom of riding on a rail-trail, welcome back! You'll find *Rail-Trails: New England* to be a useful and fun guide to your favorite trails, as well as an introduction to pathways you have yet to travel.

For readers who are discovering, for the first time, the adventures you can have on a rail-trail, thank you for joining the rail-trail movement. Since 1986, Rails-to-Trails Conservancy has been the No. 1 supporter and defender of these priceless public corridors. We are excited to bring you *Rail-Trails: New England* so you, too, can enjoy this region's rail-trails.

Built on unused, former railroad corridors, these hiking and biking trails are an ideal way to connect with your community, with nature, and with your friends and family. I've found that rail-trails have a way of bringing people together, and as you'll see from this book, there are opportunities in every state you visit to get on a trail. Whether you're looking for a place to exercise, explore, commute, or play—there is a rail-trail in this book for you.

So I invite you to sit back, relax, pick a trail that piques your interest—and then get out, get active, and have some fun. I'll be out on the trails, too, so be sure to wave as you go by.

Happy Trails,

Keith Laughlin
President, Rails-to-Trails Conservancy

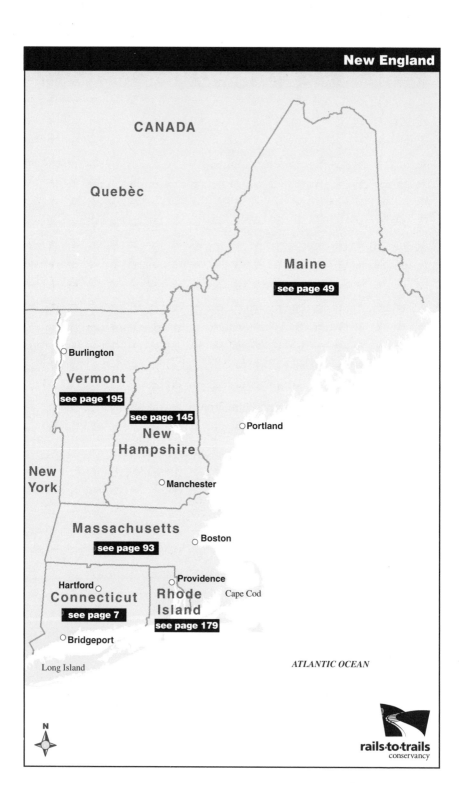

Contents

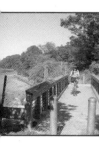

MASSACHUSETTS   93

NEW HAMPSHIRE   145

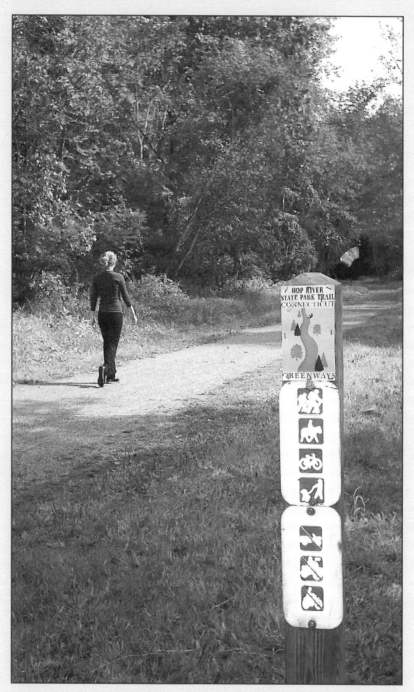

Connecticut's 15.6-mile Hop River State Park Trail

INTRODUCTION

Of the nearly 1400 rail-trails across the US, 142 thread through the New England states of Connecticut, Maine, Massachusetts, New Hampshire, Rhode Island, and Vermont. These routes relate a two-part story: The first speaks to the early years of railroading, while the second showcases efforts by Rails-to-Trails Conservancy, other groups, and their supporters to resurrect these unused railroad corridors as public-use trails.

Rail-Trails: New England highlights 60 of the region's diverse trails, each serving as a window on the communities the railroad once served. Some trails delve into the particular history of an area, such as Massachusetts' Phoenix Rail Trail, named by local schoolchildren after Fort Phoenix, within sight of which the first naval battle of the American Revolution was fought in 1775. Other trails reveal New England's industrial past, such as Rhode Island's Blackstone River Bikeway, which alternately parallels or follows the towpath of an extant historic canal along the river past 19th century textile mill villages.

Connecticut's signature trail and a key interstate link, the Farmington Canal Heritage Trail traces the route of the long-defunct canal, which once stretched from New Haven to Northampton, Massachusetts. More than 40 miles of the planned 60-mile path are now open to trail users. Another favorite, the Air Line State Park Trail, crosses streams, brooks, and the Blackledge River, as well as a pair of dramatically engineered viaducts, each more than 1000 feet long.

Rail-trails in Maine are as varied as you might expect in a state this broad, ranging from Portland's sophisticated Eastern Promenade Trail, a rail-with-trail to routes that delve into the Aroostook County wilderness, where a moose may be your only companion on more than 100 miles of trails.

Expect a similar spectrum of experiences on New Hampshire's trails, from the first few completed miles of the Cotton Valley Rail-Trail in Wolfeboro, America's oldest summer resort, to the deep woods and beaver bogs along the Rockingham Recreational Trail. White Mountain National Forest provides both hikers and bikers with challenging and scenic routes, including the Ethan Pond and Thoreau Falls trails, honoring the naturalists who helped protect this once actively logged wilderness.

Winding through farmland and rolling hills, with the Green Mountains as a serene backdrop, Vermont's rail-trails invite you to immerse yourself in the simple rural lifestyle its residents embrace. Tracing Burlington's charming waterfront en route to views of the Adirondacks across Lake Champlain, the Island Line Trail is the state's must-see trail.

No matter which route in *Rail-Trails: New England* you decide to ply, you'll be touching on the heart of the community that helped build it and the history that first brought the rails to the region. Rhode Island leads the region in trail network creation, with Providence as its hub. Check out the stunning views of Narragansett Bay along the East Bay Bicycle Path, the state's first rail-trail.

What is a Rail-Trail?

Rail-trails are multiuse public paths built along former railroad corridors. Most often flat or following a gentle grade, they are suited to walking, running, cycling, mountain biking, inline skating, cross-country skiing, horseback riding, and wheelchair use. Since the 1960s, Americans have created more than 13,000 miles of rail-trails throughout the country.

These extremely popular recreation and transportation corridors traverse urban, suburban, and rural landscapes. Many preserve historic landmarks, while others serve as wildlife conservation corridors, linking isolated parks and establishing greenways in developed areas. Rail-trails also stimulate local economies by boosting tourism and promoting trailside businesses.

What is a Rail-with-Trail?

A rail-with-trail is a public path that parallels a still-active rail line. Some run adjacent to high-speed, scheduled trains, often linking public transportation stations, while others follow tourist routes and slow-moving excursion trains. Many share an easement, separated from the rails by extensive fencing. There are more than 115 rails-with-trails in the US.

HOW TO USE THIS BOOK

*R*ail-Trails: New England provides the information you'll need to plan a rewarding rail-trail trek. With words to inspire you and maps to chart your path, it makes choosing the best route a breeze. Following are some of the highlights.

Maps

You'll find three levels of maps in this book: an **overall regional map**, **state locator maps**, and **detailed trail maps**.

The New England region includes Connecticut, Maine, Massachusetts, New Hampshire, Rhode Island, and Vermont. Each chapter details a particular state's network of trails, marked on locator maps in the chapter introduction. Use these maps to find the trails nearest you, or select several neighboring trails and plan a weekend hiking or biking excursion. Once you find a trail on a state locator map, simply flip to the corresponding page number for a full description. Accompanying trail maps mark each route's access roads, trailheads, parking areas, restrooms, and other defining features.

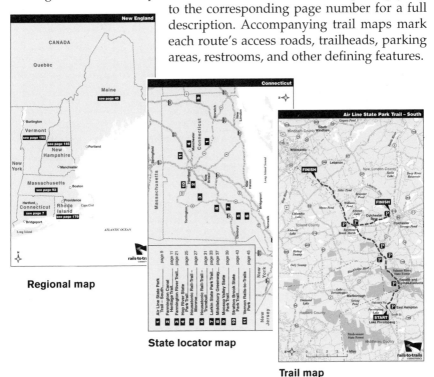

Regional map

State locator map

Trail map

3

Trail Descriptions

Trails are listed in alphabetical order within each chapter. Each description leads off with a set of summary information, including trail endpoints and mileage, a roughness index, the trail surface, and possible uses.

The map and summary information list the trail endpoints (either a city, street, or more specific location), with suggested points from which to start and finish. Additional access points are marked on the maps and mentioned in the trail descriptions. The maps and descriptions also highlight available amenities, including parking and restrooms, as well as such area attractions as shops, services, museums, parks, and stadiums. Trail length is listed in miles.

Each trail bears a roughness index rating from 1 to 3. A rating of 1 indicates a smooth, level surface that is accessible to users of all ages and abilities. A 2 rating means the surface may be loose and/or uneven and could pose a problem for road bikes and wheelchairs. A 3 rating suggests a rough surface that is only recommended for mountain bikers and hikers. Surfaces can range from asphalt or concrete to ballast, cinder, crushed stone, gravel, grass, dirt, and/or sand. Where relevant, trail descriptions address alternating surface conditions.

All rail-trails are open to pedestrians, and most allow bicycles, except where noted in the trail summary or description. The summary also indicates wheelchair access. Other possible uses include inline skating, mountain biking, hiking, horseback riding, fishing, and cross-country skiing. While most trails are off-limits to motor vehicles, some local trail organizations do allow ATVs and snowmobiles.

Trail descriptions themselves suggest an ideal itinerary for each route, including the best parking areas and access points, where to begin, your direction of travel, and any highlights along the way. The text notes any connecting or neighboring routes, with page numbers for the respective trail descriptions. Following each description are directions to the recommended trailheads.

Each trail description also lists a local contact (name, address, phone number, and website) for further information. Be sure to call these trail managers or volunteer groups in advance for updates and current conditions.

Key to Map Icons

Parking

Drinking water

Bathrooms

Trail Use

Rail-trails are popular routes for a range of uses, often making them busy places to play. Trail etiquette applies. If passing other trail users on your bicycle, always try to pass on the left with an audible warning such as a bike-mounted bell or a polite but firm, "Passing on your left!" For your safety and that of other trail users, keep children and pets from straying into oncoming trail traffic. Keep dogs leashed, and supervise children until they can demonstrate proper behavior.

Cyclists and inline skaters should wear helmets, reflective clothing, and other safety gear, as some trails involve hazardous road crossings. It's also best to bring a flashlight or bike- or helmet-mounted light for tunnel passages or twilight excursions.

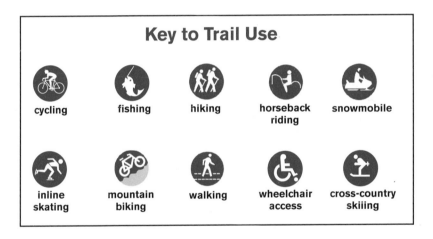

Key to Trail Use

cycling	fishing	hiking	horseback riding	snowmobile
inline skating	mountain biking	walking	wheelchair access	cross-country skiing

Learn More

While *Rail-Trails: New England* is a helpful guide to available routes in the region, it wasn't feasible to list every rail-trail in New England, and new rail-trails spring up each year. To learn about additional rail-trails in your area or to plan a trip to an area beyond the scope of this book, log on to the Rails-to-Trails Conservancy home page (www.railstotrails.org) and click on the Find a Trail link. RTC's online database lists more than 1400 rail-trails nationwide, searchable by state, county, city, trail name, surface type, length, activity, and/or keywords regarding your interest. A number of listings include photos and reviews from people who've already visited the trail.

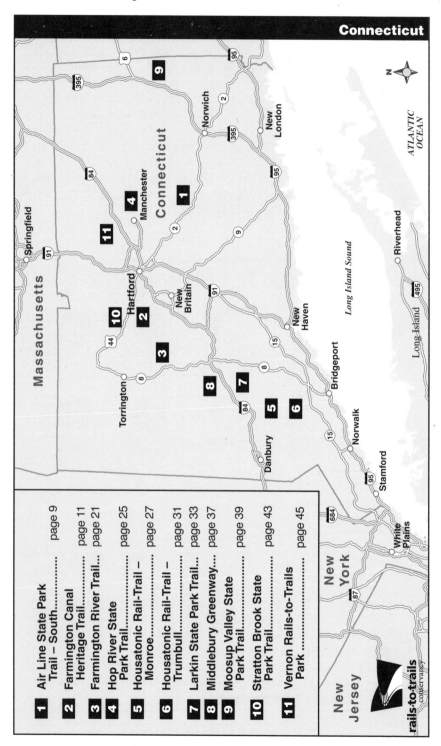

Connecticut

ATLANTIC OCEAN

Long Island Sound

Long Island

Massachusetts

Connecticut

New York

New Jersey

Springfield
Norwich
New London
Manchester
Hartford
New Britain
New Haven
Torrington
Bridgeport
Danbury
Norwalk
Stamford
White Plains
Riverhead

rails-to-trails conservancy

Connecticut

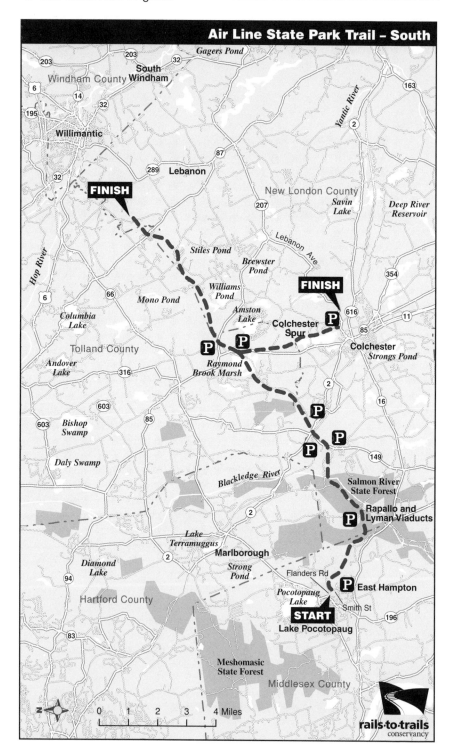

Air Line State Park Trail – South

Air Line State Park Trail – South

Air Line State Park Trail showcases the engineering behind the Air Line Railroad, laid down through this hilly region in 1873 as a direct route between Boston and New York. As its name implies, the tracks ran flat and straight, like "a line in the air." The Air Line employed the finest trains of the day, featuring the Pullman Palace Car, marketed as the "White Train" for its luxurious white-and-gold decor.

Frequent rider Rudyard Kipling once wrote of the line:

Without a jar, or roll, or antic
Without a stop to Willimantic …
Rain nor snow ne'er stops its flight
It makes New York at nine each night

The south section of the trail stretches from East Hampton to Willimantic, linking midway with a spur south to Colchester. Once completed, the route will run from East Hampton all the way to Rhode Island, where it will connect with the Blackstone River Bikeway (see page 181). If this open stretch is a glimpse of things to come, it will be a premier trail, and Willimantic could

Location
Hartford, Middlesex, New London, and Windham counties

Endpoints
East Hampton, Colchester, and Windham

Mileage
22.4

Roughness Index
2

Surface
Crushed stone

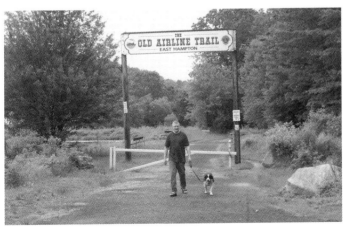

This trail (and its namesake Air Line Railroad) gets its name from the notion that the fastest route between Boston and New York would be "a line in the air."

become a trail hub, offering connections to the Hop River and Moosup Valley state park trails (see pages 25 and 39, respectively).

Round-trip riders should start in East Hampton. If you forgot to fill your water bottle at home, you can do so in the first half mile from one of the small waterfalls, created when railroad crews blasted "Bishops Cut" through solid rock.

Over the next 3 miles, you'll cross the Rapallo and Lyman Viaducts. Built in the 1870s, each spans more than a thousand feet, the latter soaring more than 150 feet above the valley floor. In 1913, crews reinforced the viaducts with rock and sediment to support heavier trains. Visible from trailside benches, the top corner of each span pokes out through the fill.

The onward trail soars over boisterous, rushing streams, smaller brooks, and the broad Blackledge River before crossing a causeway through Raymond Brook Marsh. Watch for signs of beaver.

An eighth of a mile from a trailhead and large parking area on State Route 85, the 3.4-mile Colchester Spur Rail-Trail joins the main line. Though a tad rougher, the spur offers an enjoyable ride through hemlock woods. You'll soon cross 85 and eventually emerge at an undeveloped trailhead anchored by the old Colchester Railroad Station and its twin depots.

While you can continue on the Air Line several miles, the trail becomes rougher and less defined and lacks a formal trailhead.

DIRECTIONS

To reach the western trailhead in East Hampton, take State Route 2 to Exit 13 and follow State Route 66 south for 4 miles. Turn left on State Route 196/Lakeview Street and drive a half mile, then turn left on Flanders Road and drive a quarter mile. Turn right on Smith Street; the trailhead is on the left.

The best eastern trailhead is at the junction of state routes 207 and 85 in Colchester. Take Route 2 to Exit 18, follow State Route 16 for a half mile, then turn left on Route 85. The parking lot is 4 miles down on the left.

Contact: Connecticut Department of Environmental Protection
79 Elm Street
Hartford, CT 06106
(860) 424-3200

Farmington Canal Heritage Trail

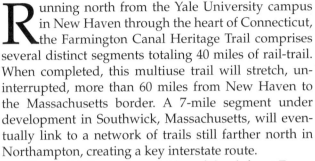

Running north from the Yale University campus in New Haven through the heart of Connecticut, the Farmington Canal Heritage Trail comprises several distinct segments totaling 40 miles of rail-trail. When completed, this multiuse trail will stretch, uninterrupted, more than 60 miles from New Haven to the Massachusetts border. A 7-mile segment under development in Southwick, Massachusetts, will eventually link to a network of trails still farther north in Northampton, creating a key interstate route.

The trail follows the corridor of the defunct Farmington Canal, New England's onetime longest canal. Completed in 1835, the waterway stretched 87 miles from New Haven to Northampton, boasting 28 locks and three aqueducts. While it was an engineering marvel, the canal was never profitable, and in 1848, the Farmington Canal Railroad (a.k.a. New Haven & Northampton Railroad) acquired the right-of-way and filled in much of the channel to make way for the tracks. (The rail line met a similar fate in the 1980s.) Traces of the canal remain throughout the Farmington Valley. Most notable is Lock 12, a trailside museum in Cheshire that centers on the restored lock. To date, the rail-trail spans the following four segments: New Haven, Hamden to Cheshire, Southington, and Farmington to the Massachusetts border.

Location
New Haven and Hartford counties

Endpoints
New Haven, Hamden to Cheshire, Southington, Farmington to Massachusetts border

Mileage
40

Roughness Index
1

Surface
Asphalt, crushed stone

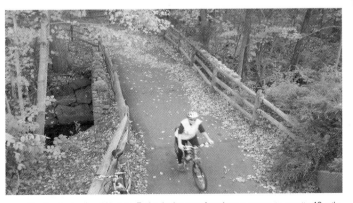

The Farmington Canal Heritage Trail is broken into four distinct segments over its 40-mile course.

11

Farmington Canal Heritage Trail

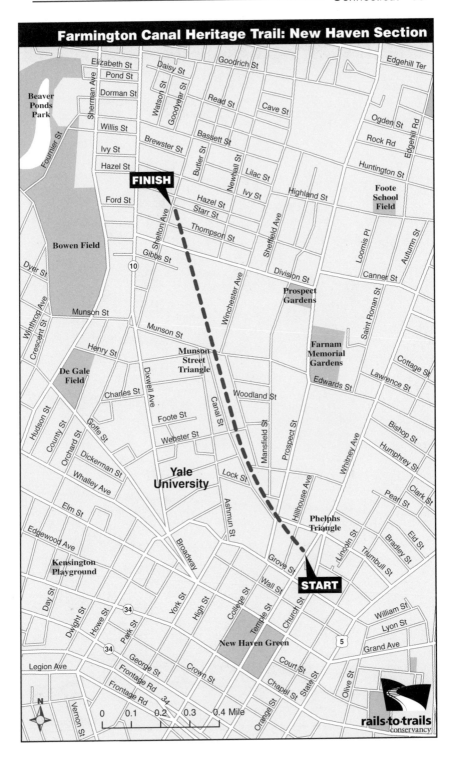

Farmington Canal Heritage Trail: New Haven Section

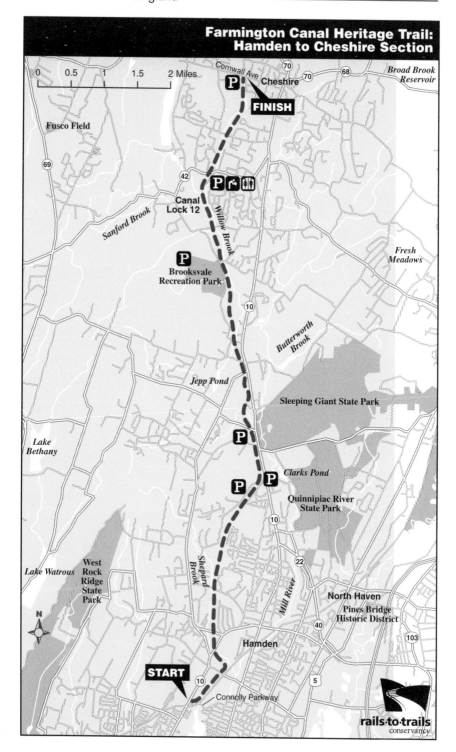

**Farmington Canal Heritage Trail:
Hamden to Cheshire Section**

New Haven Section

Anchoring the trail's southern terminus is Yale's new Malone Engineering Building, designed by prominent architect Caesar Pelli. A landscaped setting and reproduced streetlamps lend atmosphere to this 1.25-mile, asphalt-paved, urban path. There is no designated trail parking, but on-street or garage parking is available. Starr Street marks the trail's end.

DIRECTIONS

To reach the southern trailhead on the Yale campus, take Interstate 91 to Exit 3/Trumbull Street. Drive straight on Trumbull for three blocks to Hillhouse Avenue and look for on-street or garage parking. On weekends and after 4:30 p.m. on weekdays, Yale's parking lots are open to the public for free.

To continue to the Hamden to Cheshire section by bike, riders need to travel 4 miles on lightly trafficked roads. Turn right on Starr, travel one block, turn left on Newhall Street, and continue about a mile through the Putnam Avenue intersection; Newhall becomes Leeder Hill Drive. Follow Leeder Hill to the road's end at Treadwell Street, take a right, then take an immediate left on Martin Terrace. At the road's end, turn left on Mather Street, followed by a right on Waite Street. (You'll pass a series of lakes on water company property.) Take the first left on Coram Street, then left again on Beverly Road. Follow Beverly around, then bear right on Woodbine Street, skirting the water company property. Make the third left on Elgin Street, go one block, then continue straight on Connolly Parkway. At Wilbur Cross Parkway (State Route 15), turn right to pick up the Hamden to Cheshire section.

Hamden to Cheshire Section

A prominent sign for the New Haven & Northampton Railroad—The Canal Line marks the trailhead of this popular northbound segment at the Conno lly Parkway in Hamden. Woods soon line the asphalt path, and you'll cross bridge after bridge over a meandering stream. To learn about the corridor's canal and railroad roots, pause to read trailside historical markers and watch for the old brick depot and adjacent freight house just past the second parking area. Approaching Cheshire, you'll reach the aforementioned Lock 12 and keeper's

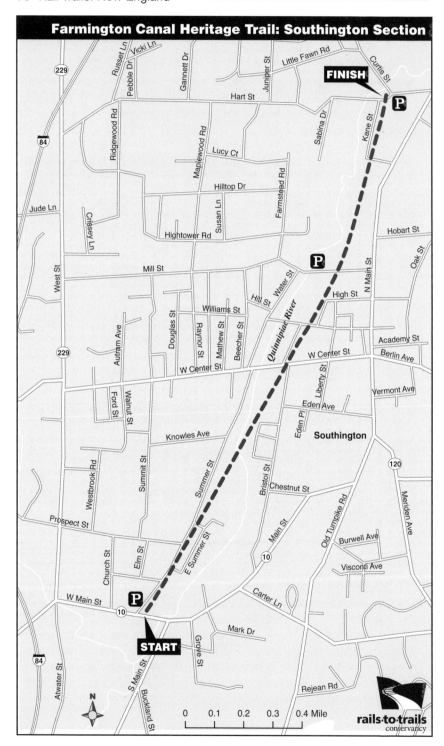

Farmington Canal Heritage Trail: Southington Section

house, now a historical park. Here you'll find trailhead parking, picnic tables, toilets, a drinking fountain, and a phone. Trail's end lies 1.6 miles north at a parking lot on Cornwall Avenue in Cheshire.

DIRECTIONS

To reach the Cheshire trailhead, take Interstate 691 to Exit 3 and head south on State Route 10/Highland Avenue through town. Turn right on Cornwall Avenue and proceed to the trailhead and adjacent parking. To drive to the southern access point, leave Route 15 (Wilbur Cross Parkway) at Exit 60 and drive north on Route 10 (Dixwell Avenue) for a quarter mile. Take the first entrance to the mall on your right and proceed to the large parking lot on the south side of the mall, which is adjacent to the trail.

Southington Section

From an inviting trailhead parking area on West Main Street in downtown Southington, this 2-mile asphalt trail bridges the Quinnipiac River and passes through the heart of a restored mill section starting at Center Street. From here, turn right on Center Street to check out the downtown eateries, or continue north to the trail's end on Hart Street.

DIRECTIONS

To reach the West Main Street trailhead, take Interstate 691 to Exit 3 and head north on State Route 10/South Main Street to West Main. Turn left on West Main and proceed to the trailhead parking area.

Farmington to the Massachusetts Border Section

Despite a few on-road detours, the 22-mile northern section of the Farmington Canal Heritage Trail is a rewarding bike ride. It shares its Tunxis Meade Park trailhead with the 8.5-mile Farmington River Trail (see page 21).

Within the first mile, pause to admire the view from a high bridge over the Farmington River. At mile 3, the Thompson Road trailhead provides restrooms. The trail first leaves the corridor 5.8 miles along in Avon, meandering a mile along surface streets and beneath Route 44 before rejoining the corridor at Sperry Park. Continue north through East Granby.

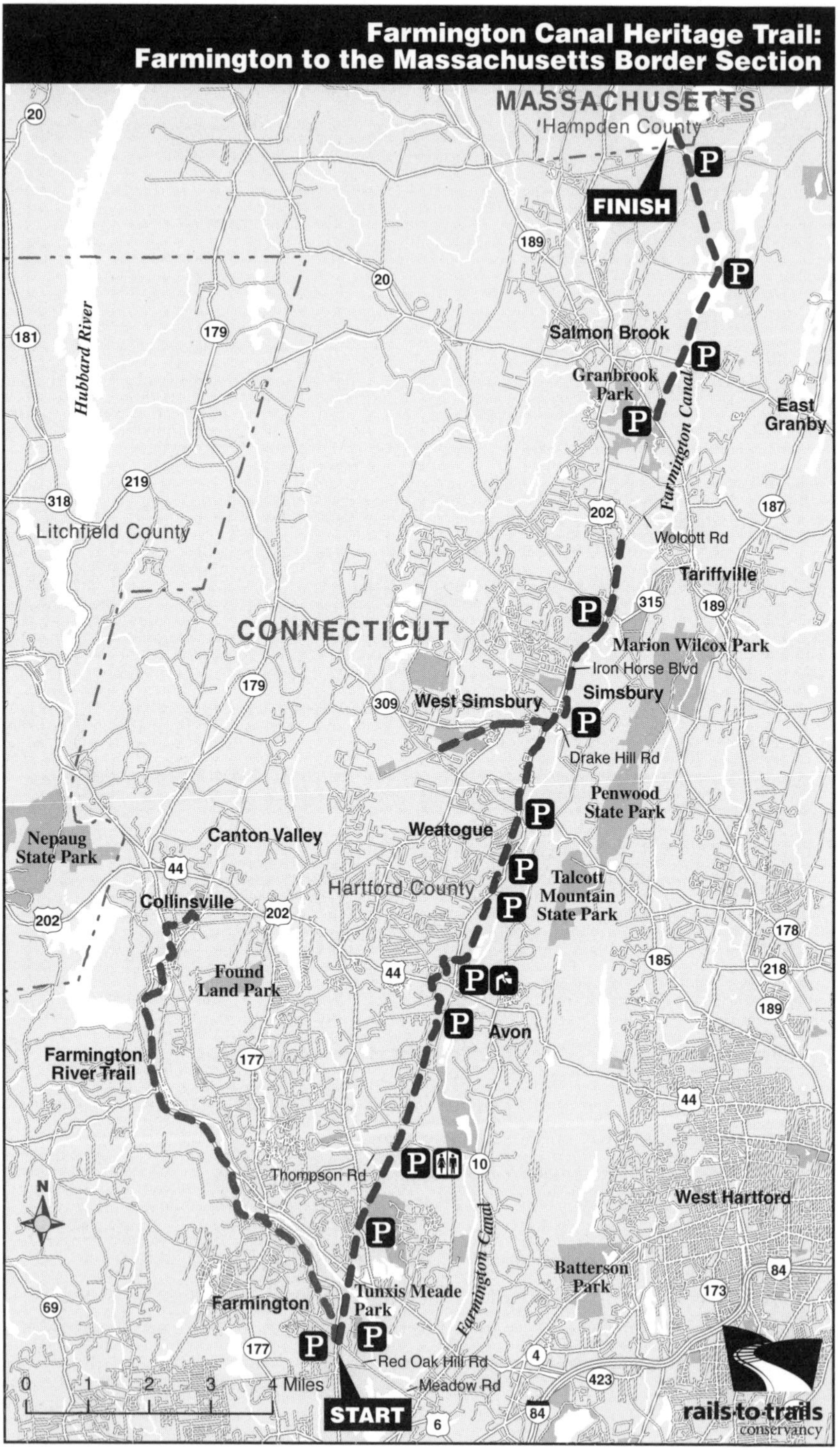

Farmington Canal Heritage Trail:
Farmington to the Massachusetts Border Section

MASSACHUSETTS
Hampden County
FINISH

Salmon Brook

Granbrook Park

East Granby

Hubbard River

Litchfield County

CONNECTICUT

Farmington Canal

Wolcott Rd

Tariffville

Marion Wilcox Park

Iron Horse Blvd

West Simsbury

Simsbury

Drake Hill Rd

Penwood State Park

Weatogue

Nepaug State Park

Canton Valley

Hartford County

Talcott Mountain State Park

Collinsville

Found Land Park

Avon

Farmington River Trail

West Hartford

Thompson Rd

Batterson Park

Farmington

Tunxis Meade Park

Red Oak Hill Rd

Meadow Rd

START

0 1 2 3 4 Miles

rails-to-trails
conservancy

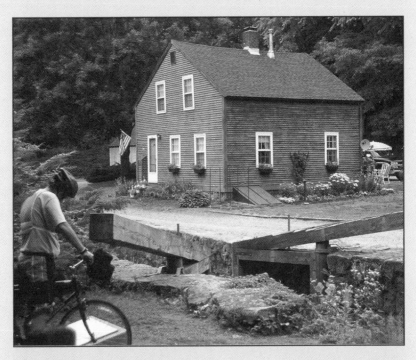

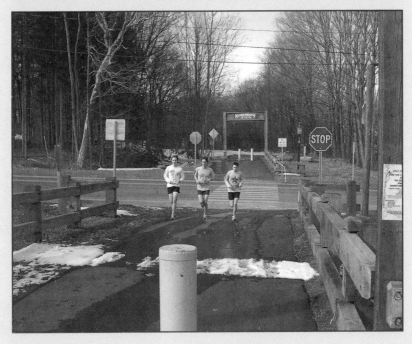

The trail passes canal locks of the defunct Farmington Canal and weaves its way through a slew of New England communities.

Approaching Simsbury, the trail passes restored brownstone buildings on the campus of aerospace and defense conglomerate Ensign-Bickford, which started in 1836 as a manufacturer of William Bickford's safety fuses for mining. Reaching a small bridge on Route 10, briefly follow the sidewalk, then turn right on Drake Hill Road and look for the trailhead to the right of Iron Horse Boulevard; turn left here to rejoin the corridor.

The trail continues north, paralleling the boulevard and passing Drake Hill Road Park. On a crisp fall day with a youth soccer game in progress, the colors of changing leaves competing with team uniforms, this stretch is a treat to travel. The trail continues 4 miles to a major break at Wolcott Road.

From here, you can either backtrack to the closest trailhead at Route 315 or, if you're a confident road cyclist, continue to the border. At Wolcott Road, turn right and travel a mile to a three-way intersection. Take another right, go about 100 yards, and turn left on Route 189. The trailhead lies a mile down this road on your right. (Note: The train depot on the left side of the road is a private home.) From here, the trail continues 4 miles to the Massachusetts border.

DIRECTIONS

To reach the southern trailhead in Farmington, take Interstate 84 to Exit 38 (from the south) or Exit 39 (from the north). Once in town, drive a mile west of Route 10 on Meadow Road to Tunxis Meade Park. (The first asphalt trail to the right of Meadow Road isn't the rail-trail, but a wonderful spur to the center of historic Farmington, whose museums and colonial architecture are worth a side trip.)

To reach the State Route 315 trailhead, take I-84 to Exit 38 (from the south) or 39 (from the north). Once in Farmington, head north on Route 10 through Avon and Simsbury. The Route 315 trailhead parking area lies 2 miles beyond the Iron Horse Boulevard trailhead.

Contact: Farmington Canal Rail-to-Trail Association
940 Whitney Avenue
Hamden, CT 06517
www.farmingtoncanal.org

Farmington River Trail

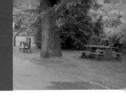

A work in progress, the Farmington River Trail offers an 8.5-mile excursion along the eponymous scenic river. Along its wilder stretches, you'll spot canoeists, kayakers, and fly-fishermen. The southern trailhead at Tunxis Meade Park in Farmington also serves as a trailhead for the Farmington Canal Heritage Trail. Be sure to follow signs to the river trail.

The trail follows the bed of the former New Haven & Northampton Railroad, originally named the Farmington Canal Railroad after the water route it supplanted, which ran from New Haven north into Massachusetts. Eventually, the river trail will stretch 18 miles north and reconnect with the Farmington Canal Heritage Trail, forming a 30-mile loop.

Two miles in, beyond its junction with State Route 177 in Unionville, the trail follows a quarter-mile road. Don't take the large bridge leading north; instead, carefully cross Route 177 at the crosswalk and head straight on Railroad Avenue. At the road's end, thread the openings in the guardrail and continue straight on the dirt path; don't turn left uphill into the new development. The trail follows the dirt path for a half mile and

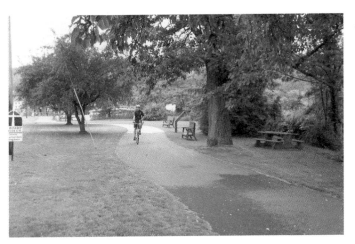

The Farmington River Trail and the Farmington Canal Heritage Trail will one day form a 30-mile loop.

Location
Hartford County

Endpoints
Farmington to Collinsville

Mileage
8.5

Roughness Index
2

Surface
Asphalt, crushed stone, cinder, dirt

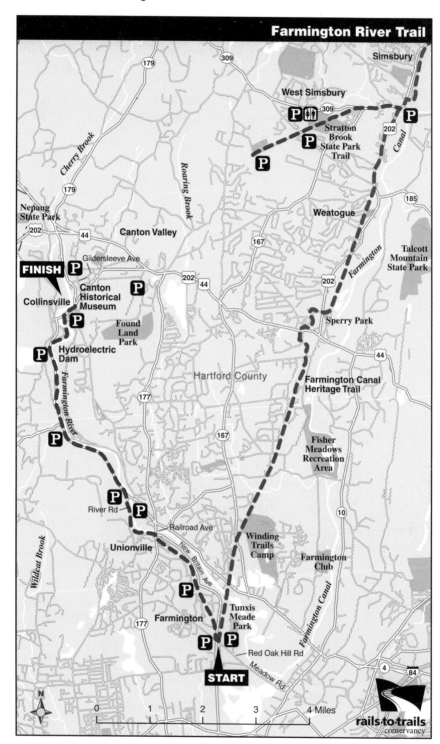

Farmington River Trail

then crosses River Road. The onward trail parallels the river on the right and Route 4 on the left, well buffered by woods.

Over the next 3 miles the trail follows the remnants of an old road and passes a defunct hydroelectric dam. Pause to read interpretive signs about this segment of the river and how it inspired several famous painters. At 7.5 miles, a ramp climbs to a restored train bridge over the river. This wonderful gateway emerges on historic Collinsville, the current end of the trail.

The trail passes the historical Collins Company mill en route to the village, which retains traces of the 19th century. Allow plenty of time to browse the Canton Historical Museum, which relates the town's history, displays an extensive collection of Victorian-era artifacts, and operates a model railroad.

DIRECTIONS

To reach the southern trailhead in Farmington, take Interstate 84 to Exit 38 and follow US Hwy. 6 west. Drive 3 miles and turn right on Route 10 north. After a quarter mile, turn left on Meadow Road and continue a mile to the parking lot at Tunxis Meade Park, on the right. From the lot, take the sidewalk along Red Oak Hill Road for 100 yards, turn right, and cross New Britain Avenue to the trailhead.

To reach the northern trailhead, take US Hwy. 44 to State Route 179 south. Collinsville lies a mile from this junction. Just before town, turn right on Gildersleeve Avenue, where the trail follows a boardwalk along the river. You'll find limited roadside parking here and additional parking in town.

Contact: Farmington Valley Trails Council
PO Box 576
Tariffville, CT 06081
(860) 658-4065

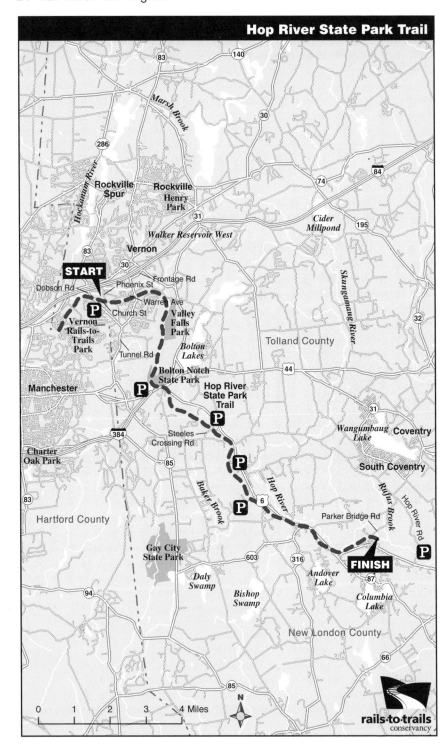

Hop River State Park Trail

Hop River State Park Trail

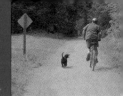

Hop River State Park Trail is one of Connecticut's top rail-trails. Narrow cuts and a lush tree canopy make for enjoyable visits all year. Most of the 15.6-mile route from the Manchester/Vernon town line to Hop River Road follows a crushed stone surface. Work is underway to extend the trail east along State Route 6. Several new bridges carry the rail-trail over side roads, but be careful: Bridges under development offer few safeguards and little warning of steep drop-offs.

For an almost seamless 12-mile eastward trek, begin at the Vernon Rails-to-Trails Park on Church Street. The first few miles climb gradually past impressive rock outcrops. Beyond the Bolton Notch parking lot, the trail passes beneath State Route 44 and US Hwy. 6, threads a narrow rock cut, then descends several miles through thick woods. Past Steeles Crossing Road, US 6 comes into view on your left, but not so close as to break the mood. Keep watch for small waterfalls like the one near Burnap Brook Road.

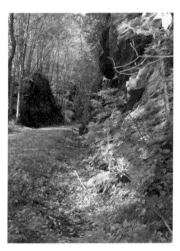

Cool cuts in the rock along the trail were made when the railroad passed through the region.

The bridge is out at State Route 316; keep back from the edge, as there's no barricade. Trail users with children are advised to turn back at this point. Others may choose to circumvent the gap and take in the next 2 miles of trail. Those cycling the trail should dismount and walk down carefully to US 6. You'll need to lift your bike over the guardrail—be sure drivers see you as they negotiate the turn onto 316.

Don't cross the road and try to climb the steep facing bank; instead, take the road to the right of the small triangular park/memorial and follow it uphill 50 yards

Location
Hartford and Tolland counties

Endpoints
Manchester/Vernon town line to Hop River Road near Columbia

Mileage
15.6

Roughness Index
2

Surface
Crushed stone, gravel, dirt

25

to rejoin the trail. A mile later, you'll pass beneath US 6 through a new, 100-foot lighted tunnel. Another mile brings you to Parker Bridge Road. This is a good place to turn around or arrange for pickup, as there's no official trail parking and the bridge to Hop River Road is out.

DIRECTIONS

The Church Street trailhead in Vernon is just 1 mile south of Interstate 84, and located between Phoenix and Washington streets. To reach the Church Street trailhead from Hartford, take I-84 east to Exit 65 and follow signs to State Route 30 north. Turn right at the first traffic signal on Dobson Road and cross beneath the interstate. Dobson becomes Washington Street. A mile south, turn left on Church Street. Trailhead parking is ahead on the left.

To reach the trailhead from Exit 66, bear right on Frontage Road, then turn left on Tunnel Road. After a quarter mile, turn right on Warren Avenue. Drive a half mile, take a left on Phoenix Street, then an immediate right on Church. Trailhead parking is on the right.

Contact: Connecticut Department
of Environmental Protection
79 Elm Street
Hartford, CT 06106
(860) 424-3200

Housatonic Rail-Trail – Monroe

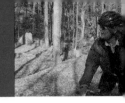

Monroe residents use this largely forested 4.3-mile section of the Housatonic (known locally as the Monroe Railbed Trail) as a convenient bike route to William E. Wolfe Park. Visiting rail-trail users also gravitate around the park, which centers on Great Hollow Lake's attractive sand beach and swimming area, restrooms, and picnic tables. Nonmotorized boating is permitted on the 16-acre lake, and a paved, pedestrian-only walking path circles its shoreline.

The Housatonic trailhead is accessible via the entrance road to the lake, just off the left shoulder at a bend in the road. You'll need to purchase a day-use sticker to park here. The rail-trail's crushed stone surface is generally compact enough even for wheelchair use.

Watch for traces of the Housatonic Railroad, one of New England's first rail lines, which carried passengers and freight between Monroe and Bridgeport. The most notable remnant is a stone-arch bridge that is on the Connecticut List of Historic Places. Also note the drill holes amid cuts blasted through solid rock for the rail corridor.

Location
Fairfield County

Endpoints
Monroe to Newtown town line

Mileage
4.3

Roughness Index
2

Surface
Crushed stone

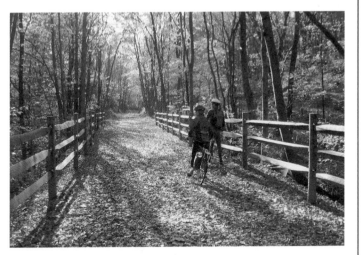

The Housatonic Rail-Trail – Monroe provides a canopy of leaves in the fall.

Housatonic Rail-Trail – Monroe

Cogers Pond

Rowledge Pond

High Bridge Rd

Avalon Way

High Rock Rd

Botsford Hill Rd

25

Swamp Rd

FINISH

Meadow Brook Rd

Fan Hill Rd

Garder Rd

Pine Tree Hill Rd

Bear Hills Rd

Lantern Dr

Lanes Mine Nature Park

Pastors Walk

Guinea Rd

Wiltan Dr

P

Pepper St

Jockey Hollow Rd

Fairmount Dr

Hillcrest Rd

Northbrook Dr

Wells Rd

Maiden Ln

Flint Ridge Rd

Horizon Ct

Bart Rd

Benedict Rd

25

Hubbell Dr

Cross Bow Ln

Meadows End Rd

Pequonnock River

Longview Rd

Elm St

Hattertown Rd

Brook St

Harvester Rd

Far Horizon Dr

Crestwood Rd

Easton Rd

Bugg Hill Rd

Senior Dr

Cross Hill Rd

Hayes St

Stanley Rd

25

William E. Wolfe Park

Great Hollow Lake

P

Monroe Turnpike

Mill River

N

Judd Rd

P

Purdy Hill Rd

START

Doc Silverstone Rd

Judd Rd

Main St

Old Newtown Rd

Cutlers Farm Rd

Partridge Dr

0   0.25   0.5   0.75   1 Mile

rails to trails
conservancy

The rail-trail crosses area roads several times and includes a short on-road detour at the stone-arch bridge near the trail midpoint. You'll veer through a residential cul-de-sac, then turn left, and follow Pepper Street for a quarter mile before rejoining the trail. At the 4-mile mark, you'll cross Pepper Street for the last time. After another quarter mile, you'll reach trail's end at a large dirt pile on the Newtown town line.

Mountain bikers looking for a little adventure can tackle another quarter mile or so of rough riding. Another option: Leave the park and head 2 miles south to pick up the Housatonic Rail-Trail – Trumbull, a 3-mile section of the same former rail corridor (see page 31).

DIRECTIONS

To reach the Wolfe Park trailhead, take Interstate 84 to Exit 11 and turn left off the ramp onto Wasserman Way. At the junction with Route 25, turn left (south) and drive about 8 miles to Old Newtown Road. Turn left on Old Newtown, right on Purdy Hill Road, then left again on Doc Silverstone Road into Wolfe Park. The trailhead is off the left side of the road just south of the parking lot. There is a day-use parking fee.

Contact: Monroe Parks & Recreation Department
7 Fan Hill Road
Monroe, CT 06468
(203) 452-5416

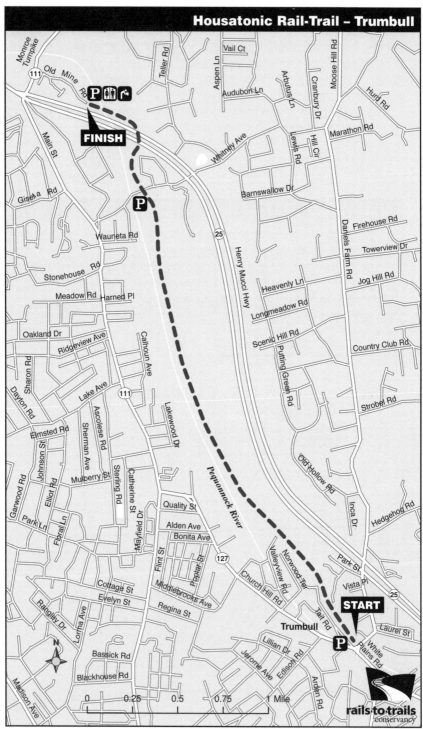

Housatonic Rail-Trail – Trumbull

Housatonic Rail-Trail – Trumbull

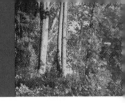

A shady respite from suburban Trumbull, this fairly flat trail overlooks the winding Pequonnock River for much of its 3.4 miles. Rapids and distinctive rock outcrops add interest. The trail begins on the railroad corridor, strays from it, then returns to emerge at Old Mine Park. The first 2.5 miles offer easy walking or cycling on dirt and gravel; the final portion is extremely rough.

Also known as Trumbull Old Mine Park Trail, this section of the Housatonic begins with a steep 20-foot climb from the road near the former town hall. Once on the trail, you quickly leave traffic noise behind as you trace hillside contours amid lush deciduous woods. Early on, the river shoots through a narrow chasm. Though you'll soon lose sight of the water, side trails descend to overlooks. Just before the first road crossing at Whitney Avenue, you'll reach a beautiful series of cascading falls and pools.

The trail crosses Whitney at a blind corner, so use caution. On the other side, the trail veers right, away from the rail corridor. This half-mile stretch to Old Mine Park is a single-track hiking trail, its surface broken by

Location
Fairfield County

Endpoints
Tait Road to Old Mine Park, Trumbull

Mileage
3.4

Roughness Index
2

Surface
Cinder, crushed stone, dirt

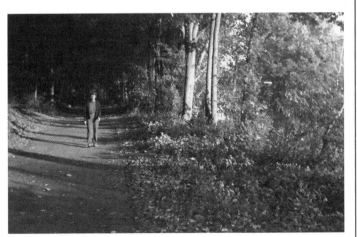

The Housatonic Rail-Trail – Trumbull offers both smooth walking and rugged hiking on its pretty path.

rocks and tree roots. Unless you're an experienced mountain biker, you'll need to walk your bike. The silence is broken only by State Route 25, which spans the trail on a bridge over the Pequonnock. Leaving the busy road behind, you'll escape once again into quiet, forested surroundings.

Old Mine Park marks the trail's northern endpoint. Here, a picturesque footbridge crosses the river to picnic tables and a pavilion with public restrooms. An interpretive sign relates the region's mining history, beginning with the Paugussett Native American tribe, which collected quartz from exposed veins for arrow points. Look for a photo of the old mine buildings following the 1855 discovery of tungsten, a metal used for hardening alloys.

If you prefer to keep moving, the park offers a multipurpose field for turf sports, as well as links to a variety of hiking trails and single-track mountain biking routes. Or you can head 2 miles north and pick up the Housatonic Rail-Trail – Monroe (see page 27), which traverses another 4 miles of this scenic railroad corridor.

DIRECTIONS

To park near the old town hall, take State Route 25 to Exit 9 and turn south on Daniel's Farm Road. At the light, take a right on State Route 127, followed by an immediate right on Tait Road (not Tait's Mill Road) to the unsigned, six-car parking area beside the old town hall (now called the Helen Plumb Building). The trailhead lies 50 yards down the road on the left.

Only permitted town residents can park at Old Mine Park; visitors may park on neighboring streets. To reach the park, take State Route 25 North to State Route 111, continue north on 111, and take the first right turn into the park. The signed trailhead is near the main parking area.

The Whitney Avenue trailhead offers a larger parking area, but only town residents and state residents with fishing licenses may purchase the required permit.

Contact: Pequonnock River Valley Park
c/o Sherwood Island State Park
PO Box 188
Green Farms, CT 06436
(203) 226-6983

Larkin State Park Trail

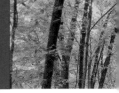

Canopied with deciduous trees for most of its 10.4 miles, the Larkin State Park Trail (a.k.a. Larkin Bridle Path) is primarily a wilderness trail, with wooded vistas, wetland views, and sparse residential development. Its railroad past began in 1881 with completion of the New York & New England Railroad between western Connecticut and New York. Following bankruptcy in 1894, the New York, New Haven, & Hartford Railroad took over the line until 1939. Dr. Charles L. Larkin purchased the corridor and gifted it to the state in 1943 for a bridle trail.

You're likely to encounter equestrians. Particularly when cycling, remember to approach horses slowly and quietly; speak softly and take your cues from their riders. You may need to stop and dismount until they pass, as horses have the right-of-way.

Typical of rail-trails in southwest Connecticut, the route plies a gentle grade across rolling topography, occasionally slicing through rock outcrops or overlooking low-lying areas. The trail's crushed stone surface is typically firm, especially in the eastern and middle portions. Surface conditions are rougher along the western

Location
New Haven County

Endpoints
Whittemore Glen State Park to Southbury

Mileage
10.4

Roughness Index
3

Surface
Gravel, cinder, crushed stone, dirt

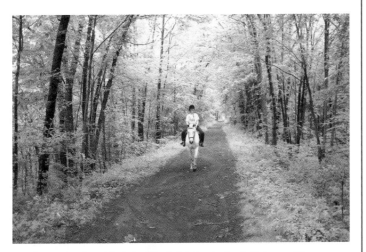

The mixed surface of the Larkin State Park Trail makes it suitable for equestrian use.

33

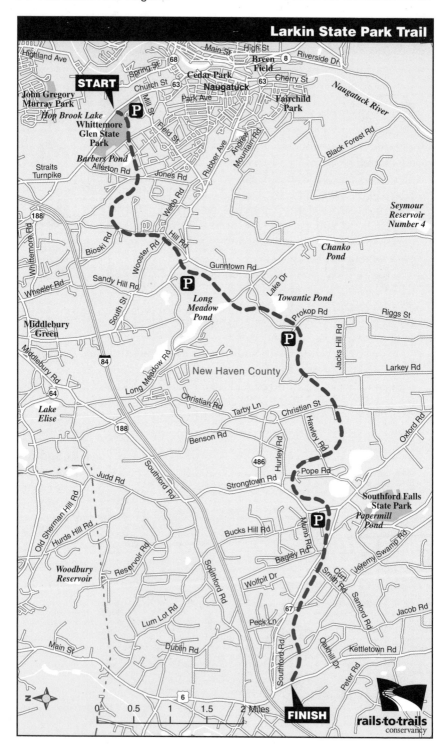

Larkin State Park Trail

section, which is rockier and somewhat eroded, making it more suitable for mountain bikes.

Near the trail midpoint at Long Meadow Road, you'll briefly leave state-owned property for a half-mile, on-road detour along a privately held stretch. Turn left on Long Meadow Road and right on Towantic Hill Road, then watch for trail access on the left side of the road. The onward trail offers lovely views of the boggy shoreline of Towantic Pond, then passes over wetlands on a causeway.

Near the west end, a short section between State Route 67 and Curt Smith Road is often very wet, and washouts persist. At some of the numerous road crossings, the trail descends or rises steeply to the road, and approaching motorists may not see you; use caution. There are no crosswalks.

DIRECTIONS

The trail parallels Interstate 84, which makes for easy trail access, although parking is limited. To reach the eastern trailhead, take I-84 to Exit 17 and head south on State Route 63. After nearly 2 miles, turn right into the small parking area for Larkin State Bridle Trail. Follow the sign to the trail.

Access from the western terminus is not a viable option, as the trail is difficult to find and there's neither parking nor even room to pull over on the shoulder. Instead, take I-84 to Exit 16 and head 2 miles south on State Route 188/Strongtown Road to a trailhead with limited parking.

Contact: South Falls State Park
Department of Environmental Protection
174 Quaker Farms Road
Southbury, CT 06488
(860) 264-5169

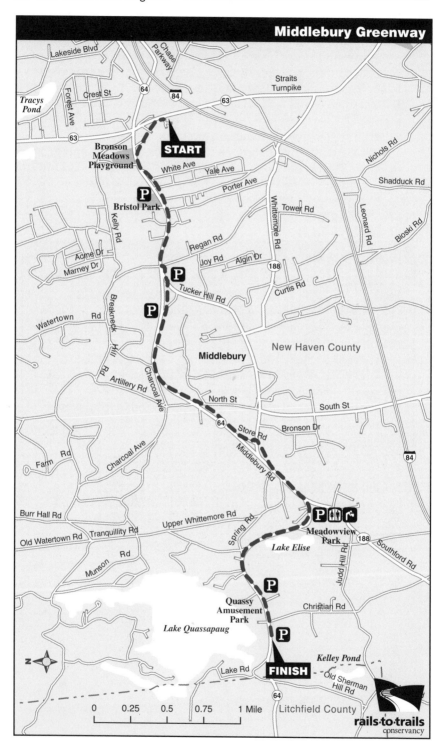

Middlebury Greenway

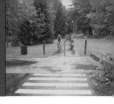

This delightful asphalt path winds 4.4 miles through the residential community of Middlebury, connecting businesses, parks, and homes. The popular trail offers residents an off-road option for running errands, and welcomes car-weary travelers on nearby Interstate 84 who wish to stretch their legs in a convenient and comfortable setting. While State Route 64 parallels the greenway for its entire length, the road won't lessen your enjoyment.

Tracing a Connecticut Company trolley line that first operated in 1908, the trail follows the contours of the land, making it hillier and more winding than a typical rail-trail. As you make your way along its route, try to imagine the open-air trolley cars bringing holidaymakers from Waterbury to Middlebury's Lake Quassapaug resorts. Unlike rail lines with a single stop in town, this state-of-the-art trolley line brought riders to the very doorstep of local homes and businesses.

If you're taking the trail out and back, travel east to west for an easier downhill return. Parking on the east end is also more convenient. The initial stretch is an in-town trail passing local businesses. You're likely to see

Location
New Haven County

Endpoints
Route 64/63 junction to Quassy Amusement Park in Middlebury

Mileage
4.4

Roughness Index
1

Surface
Asphalt

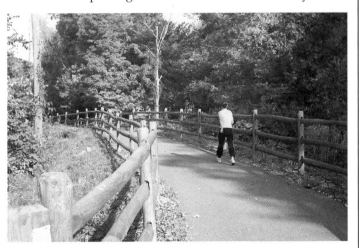

The Middlebury Greenway is a former trolley line that today takes users through neighborhoods and even an amusement park.

people running errands on foot and by bicycle. Farther west you'll come upon two small, nicely landscaped parks. Pause on a bench to catch your breath or meet a friend.

Alternating between woods and residential areas, the trail continues 2 miles to Meadowview Park, a community park with sports fields, picnic tables, a water fountain, and public restrooms. Approaching the trail's west end, you'll overlook spring-fed Lake Quassapaug and its sandy beach, and pass Quassy Amusement Park, an early destination for the trolley. The trolley closed in the 1930s when visitors began driving their cars to the resort, but the park remains popular and is known for large clam bakes and family fun. Its carousel and roller rink predate World War II.

The trail ends at an access road leading to a first-class Little League baseball field.

DIRECTIONS

To reach the eastern trailhead, take Interstate 84 to Exit 17 and follow State Route 64 west. After going through one traffic light at State Route 63 junction, you'll see a parking lot on the right. The trail starts on the other side of 64.

To reach the western terminus from I-84, take Exit 16 and follow State Route 188 north for almost 3 miles. At the junction with State Route 64, you'll see Meadowview Park on the left. You may load or unload bikes in the baseball field's parking lot, but long-term parking is not an option as the gates are sometimes locked.

Contact: Middlebury Parks & Recreation Department
1212 Whittemore Road
Middlebury, CT 06762
(203) 758-2520

Moosup Valley State Park Trail

This 5.8-mile trail is part of the planned East Coast Greenway, an off-road path that will eventually run from Calais, Maine, to Key West, Florida. Already, the Moosup Valley State Park Trail connects with rail-trails in Rhode Island that stretch from the state border about 20 miles east to Providence.

The trail follows the bed of the former New Haven Railroad, which operated this line from 1898 until 1968, when it began pulling up tracks. Wide and flat, the trail is suitable for riders of all levels, though it is not pristinely manicured. Its surface is largely hard-packed dirt, but this varies, and the trail is not recommended for road bikes. A hybrid or a mountain bike would be ideal.

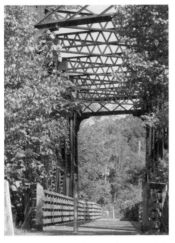

An impressive railway trestle is part of the Moosup Valley State Park Trail.

Head out on this bucolic, scenic trail, and you'll feel as though you have left civilization far behind. Much of the trail follows the Moosup River on its course past rural Moosup and Sterling on into Rhode Island. The trail begins with a large, re-decked trestle bridge. After a mile, a second bridge, as well as a dam and falls, come into view, and the trail becomes increasingly rural and wooded. You'll spot a quarry to the right, around the 2-mile point.

There's no clear line of demarcation between the end of the Moosup Valley State Park Trail and the start of the Trestle Trail, as the path is named once it enters Rhode Island. Determine your own best turnaround point.

If you plan to use the trail in autumn or early winter, be aware that hunting is popular here. In season, you're advised to wear blaze orange. (Note: Hunting is not permitted on Sundays.)

Location
Windham County

Endpoints
Moosup to Rhode Island border

Mileage
5.8

Roughness Index
2

Surface
Asphalt, ballast, crushed stone, gravel, grass, dirt, sand

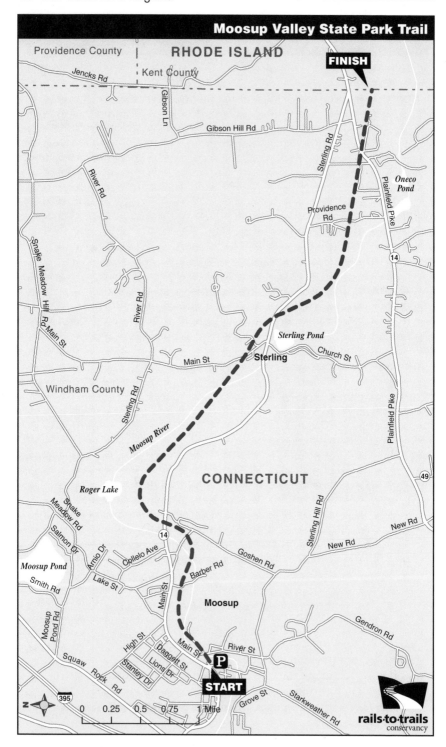

Moosup Valley State Park Trail

DIRECTIONS

To reach Moosup from Rhode Island, follow State Route 14 west from the state line; to reach it from Connecticut, take Interstate 395 to Exit 89 and follow Route 14 east toward Moosup/Sterling. The trailhead lies near the junction of Main Street/Route 14, South Main, Ward Avenue, and Prospect Street (also Route 14). It begins at the large railroad trestle on dead-end Village Center Circle, on the same side of the street as the river. Park at the Moosup Adult Learning Lab.

Contact: Eastern Division Headquarters
Department of Environmental Protection
209 Hebron Road
Marlborough, CT 06447
(860) 295-9523

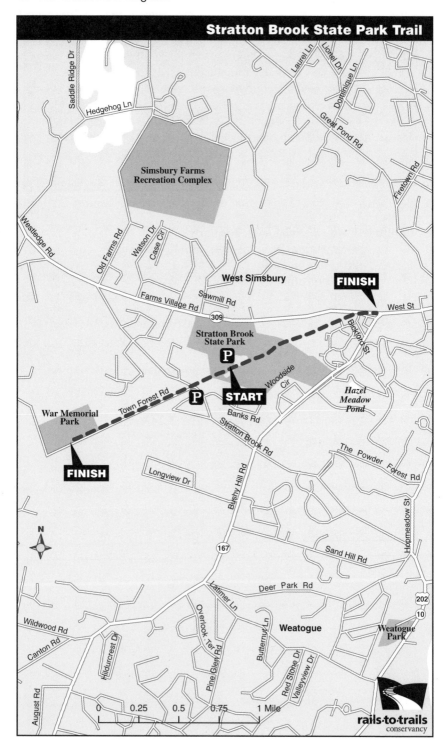

Stratton Brook State Park Trail

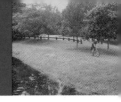

This 2-mile trail presents a great way to work up an appetite for a picnic at Stratton Brook State Park, the first state park in Connecticut to be entirely wheelchair-accessible. The park also offers picnic areas, as well as fishing and swimming on its lake, created by the Civilian Conservation Corps during the Great Depression, when it dammed the brook. A covered bridge accesses the trail midpoint.

From the covered bridge, the shaded rail-trail shoots northeast and southwest along the right-of-way of the former Connecticut Western Railroad. Head northeast to take in a mile of dense evergreen forest fragrant with pine and hemlock. Ferns carpet the forest floor, and the tree canopy creates a tunnel effect—especially beautiful in winter. After bridging Stratton Brook and rounding a gentle bend, the trail exits the park, ending at the Bushy Hill Road/State Route 309 intersection.

The trail will eventually become part of Farmington River Trail (see page 21), which links up with the longer Farmington Canal Heritage Trail (see page 11). In the meantime, you can access the canal trail by turning right on State Route 309 and following the shoulder a half mile.

Location
Hartford County

Endpoints
Stratton Brook State Park to Simsbury

Mileage
2

Roughness Index
2

Surface
Asphalt, cinder, crushed stone

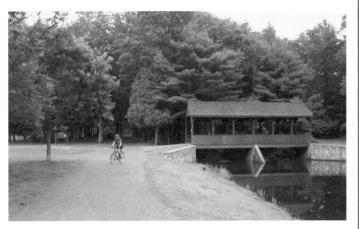

A covered bridge spans Stratton Brook at the midpoint on the Stratton Brook State Park Trail.

For a slightly longer ride or walk, turn southwest from the covered bridge and cross Stratton Brook Road. From there, the old railroad grade is a paved but seldom used road for 1.7 miles, where it enters Massacoe State Forest. Crews once used this corridor to demonstrate fire-control techniques along rail lines.

DIRECTIONS

To reach Stratton Brook State Park, take Interstate 84 to Exit 50, follow US Hwy. 44 west for 9.5 miles, then turn right on State Route 10/US Hwy. 202 north to Simsbury. From town, head south on State Route 167/Bushy Hill Road, then veer west on State Route 309 for 0.9 mile. The park entrance is on the left.

Contact: Simsbury Parks & Recreation
933 Hopmeadow Street
Simsbury, CT 06070
(860) 658-3255

Vernon Rails-to-Trails Park

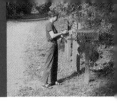

Thanks to skilled engineers with the former Hartford, Providence, & Fishkill Railroad, this pretty trail network overlooks ravines and streams and passes between rock walls verdant with ferns and lichen. Crossing a wooded terrain of hills and wetlands, it also provides a wonderful introduction to Vernon's varied neighborhoods. You may spot deer, and you'll surely notice the line of railroad-era telephone poles amid the trees. The Connecticut Army National Guard laid down the stone dust surface as a training exercise.

From the main trailhead hub on Church Street, the Vernon Rails-to-Trails Park offers three trail segments.

Stretching west and then south, a 1.8-mile spur of the Hop River State Park Trail leads to the Manchester/Vernon town line. There is no formal trailhead at the end. The park also claims a 3.9-mile eastbound stretch of the Hop River State Park Trail. From Church Street, you'll quickly pass the turnoff for the Rockville Spur on your left. The first mile links residential neighborhoods. Beyond Tunnel Road, the Vernon section of the trail leads through thick woods to the Bolton town line.

Location
Tolland County

Endpoints
Manchester/Vernon town line, Rockville, and Bolton town line

Mileage
9.7

Roughness Index
2

Surface
Crushed stone

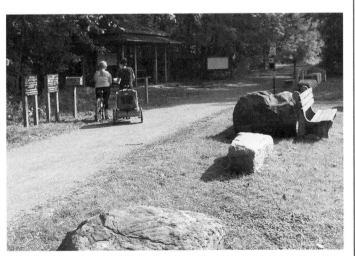

This trail offers three offshoots: the Vernon Rails-to-Trails Park, the Hop River State Park Trail, and the Rockville Spur.

45

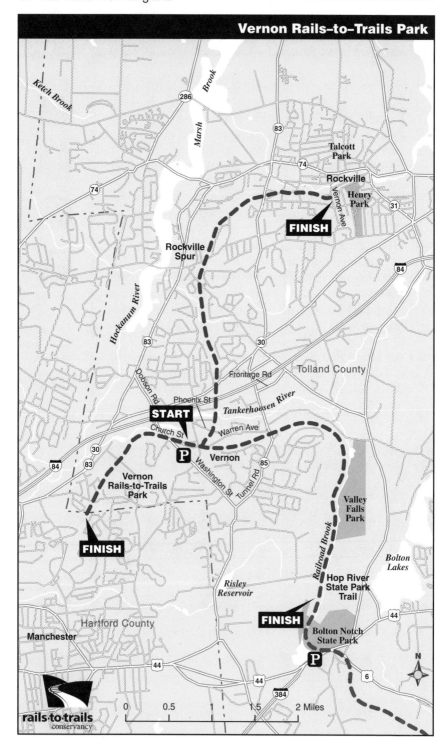

Vernon Rails–to–Trails Park

Ketch Brook

Marsh Brook

286

83

74

Talcott Park

74

Rockville

Henry Park

31

74

Rockville Spur

FINISH

Vernon Ave

84

Hockanum River

83

30

Frontage Rd

Tolland County

Dobson Rd

Phoenix St

Tankerhoosen River

START

Church St

Warren Ave

P

Vernon

85

84

30

83

Washington St

Tunnel Rd

Vernon Rails-to-Trails Park

Valley Falls Park

Bolton Lakes

FINISH

Railroad Brook

Hop River State Park Trail

Risley Reservoir

44

FINISH

Bolton Notch State Park

Hartford County

Manchester

P

6

44

44

N

384

rails·to·trails
conservancy

0   0.5   1   1.5   2 Miles

(See page 25 for the onward trail description of the Hop River State Park Trail.)

The 4-mile Rockville Spur negotiates a varied surface, sharing a sidewalk early on and crossing several roads. A half mile from the turnoff, you'll reach a trail highlight: a bridge crossing of the Tankerhoosen River. Just shy of Vernon Avenue, the spur comes to an abrupt halt at a large earthen mound atop an old bridge abutment.

At this point, you can either backtrack or (if you're on a bike) dismount, carefully descend a 50-foot embankment to the left of the abutment, and consider exploring Rockville's surface roads.

DIRECTIONS

The Vernon Rails-to-Trails Park is on Church Street between Phoenix and Washington streets, a mile south of Interstate 84. From Hartford, take I-84 east to Exit 65 and follow signs to State Route 30 north. Turn right at the first traffic signal on Dobson Road and cross beneath the interstate. Dobson becomes Washington Street. A mile south, turn left on Church Street. Trailhead parking is ahead on the left.

To reach the trailhead from Exit 66, bear right on Frontage Road, then turn left on Tunnel Road. After a quarter mile, turn right on Warren Avenue. Drive a half mile, take a left on Phoenix Street, then take an immediate right on Church Street. Trailhead parking is on the right.

Contact: Vernon Parks & Recreation
120 South Street
Vernon, CT 06066
(860) 870-3520

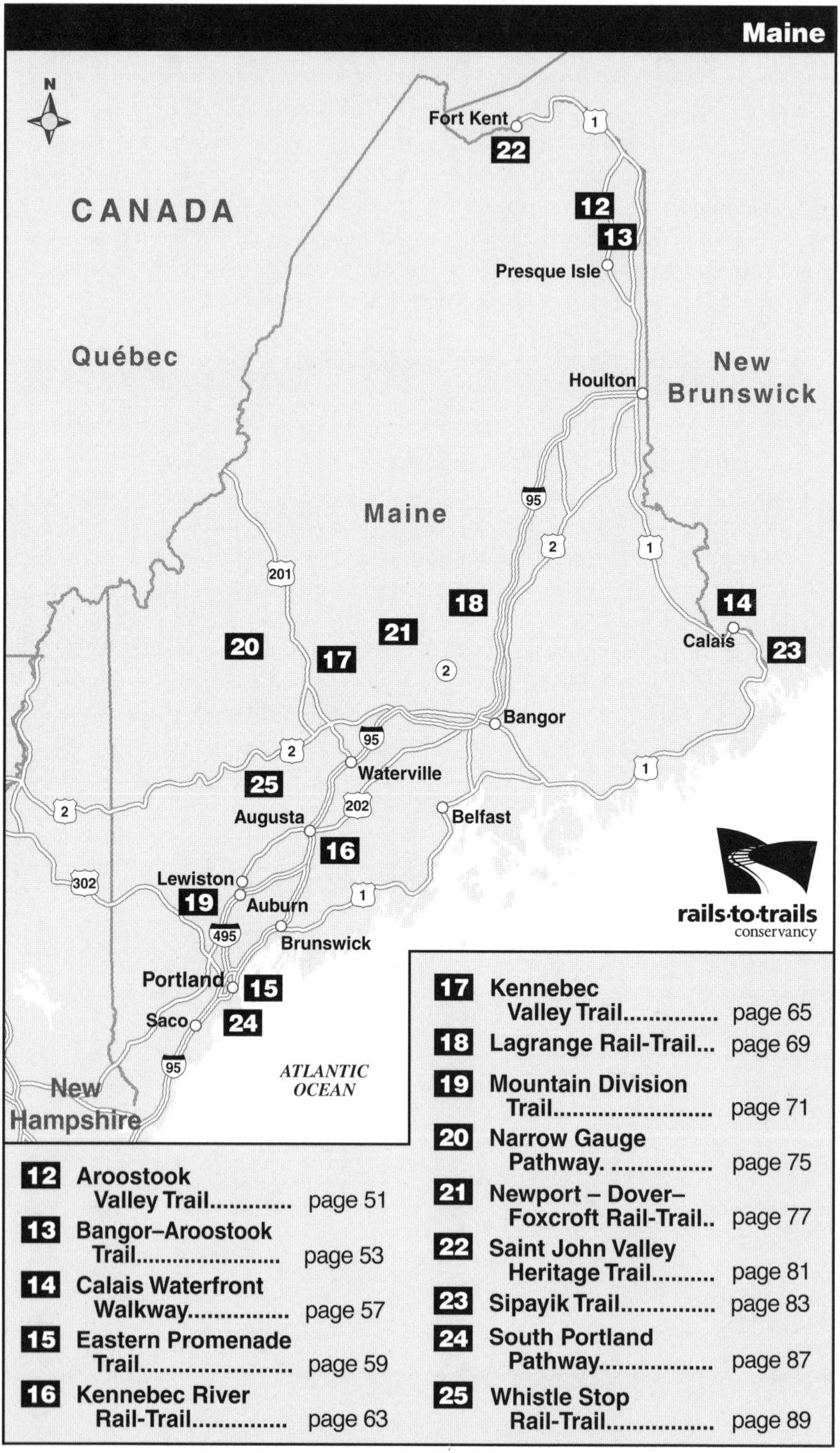

N

C A N A D A

Fort Kent

22

1

12

13

Presque Isle

Québec

New Brunswick

Houlton

95

Maine

2

1

201

18

21

14

20

17

Calais **23**

2

Bangor

2

95

Waterville

1

25

Augusta

202

Belfast

16

302

Lewiston

1

19

Auburn

495

Brunswick

Portland **15**

Saco **24**

95

ATLANTIC
OCEAN

New Hampshire

rails·to·trails
conservancy

Maine

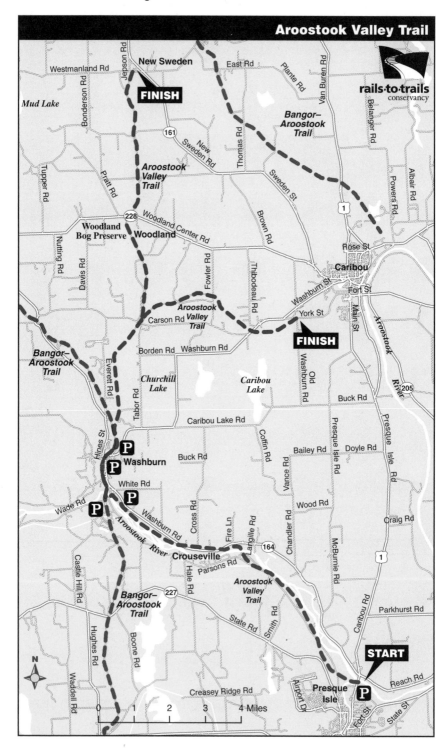

Aroostook Valley Trail

rails·to·trails
conservancy

Aroostook Valley Trail

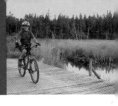

In the far northeast reaches of Maine, the Aroostook Valley Trail runs atop the bed of Aroostook County's only electric railroad, a line once used to transport passengers to school and work and to haul potatoes from farmland to market. Today the county remains a largely agricultural area, renowned for its broccoli and potatoes. The rail corridor was abandoned in 1951, and trail development began in 1994.

The 27-mile, crushed-stone rail-trail connects to the 58-mile Bangor–Aroostook Trail (see page 53), so you can opt for a short jaunt or fill up an entire day (or two) touring and exploring the region. The trails are part of northern Maine's Interconnected Trail System, which comprises more than 3000 miles of ATV and snowmobile track. Don't let the motorized users deter you: As on many of Maine's trails, the snowmobilers and ATV users here mingle peacefully with bicyclists, walkers, skiers, and dogsledders.

Whatever your mode of travel, it's easy to plan a multiday excursion. Food and lodging are readily available along the route, and signs posted at major trail

Location
Aroostook County

Endpoints
Presque Isle, New Sweden, and Caribou

Mileage
27

Roughness Index
3

Surface
Crushed stone, dirt

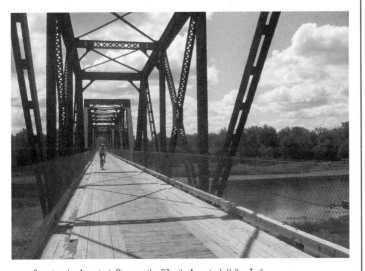

Crossing the Aroostook River on the 27-mile Aroostook Valley Trail.

intersections indicate the distance not just to the next town, but to the next meal.

Washburn marks the junction with the Bangor–Aroostook Trail. A few miles north, the Aroostook Valley Trail splits; head north toward New Sweden for a snack from the general store or east toward Caribou for food and lodging.

North of Washburn, evergreens and deciduous trees canopy the route, and wild apples hang for the picking. Elsewhere, the raised trail bisects wetland bogs, including Woodland Bog Preserve, where birders have identified 80 distinct species. Also keep watch for roaming moose and the mud-and-stick walls of beaver dams.

South of Washburn, the landscape opens up to vast potato farms. In late summer, the sweet aroma of potato blossoms fills the air. Potatoes are harvested in September and stored in potato houses—at major crossroads and abandoned sidings—until the spuds are sent to market. Watch for farm machinery crossing the trail during harvest.

DIRECTIONS

In Washburn, you'll find trailhead parking north of town at Mill Pond Park on Station Road. In Presque Isle, you'll find parking on US Hwy. 1 just north of the Aroostook Centre Mall, on the south bank of the Aroostook River.

To reach the New Sweden trailhead from Caribou, take State Route 161 about 8 miles north to New Sweden and turn left on Westmanland Road. The trailhead is at the intersection of Westmanland and Jepson roads.

Contact: Caribou Parks & Recreation
55 Bennett Drive
Caribou, ME 04736
(207) 493-4224
www.caribourec.org

Bangor–Aroostook Trail

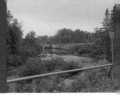

A multiuse trail shared with ATVs and snowmobiles, the 58-mile Bangor–Aroostook Trail (a.k.a. BAT) is part of northern Maine's amazing, complex Interconnected Trail System. You can easily coordinate a multiday tour on this and other area rail-trails, taking advantage of lodging and food options in towns along the way. However, sections of the BAT do lead through wilderness areas, so plan accordingly. Carry a tool kit (if biking), layered clothing, and plenty of water. Also note that although the Bangor–Aroostook Trail map indicates distinct segments of trail, there are generally connections between the endpoints that are part of this greater trail system, be they on-road segments, snowmobile trails, or less-groomed pathways.

Trains once hauled lumber and potatoes down this route to distribution centers along the East Coast. Threading a wider corridor than the connecting Aroostook Valley Trail (see page 51), the BAT crosses acres of farmland, as well as woods and wetland bogs, and it is an excellent platform for spotting a range of wildlife.

Location
Aroostook County

Endpoints
Caribou, Van Buren, Houlton, Phair, and Mapleton

Mileage
58

Roughness Index
3

Surface
Crushed stone, dirt

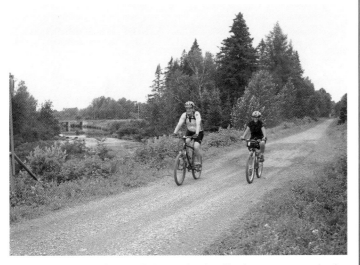

The 58-mile Bangor–Aroostook Trail is part of northern Maine's vast interconnected trail system.

53

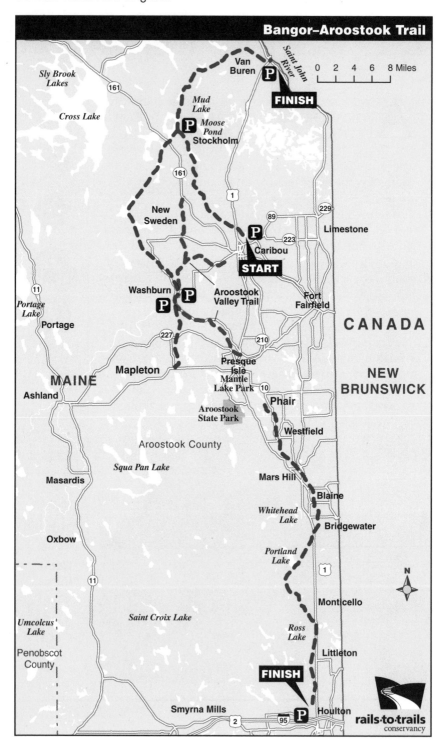

Bangor–Aroostook Trail

The best access point to this trail system is Caribou, where you'll find plenty of food, lodging, and trail information.

The area north of Stockholm is largely wilderness and is a great place to spot moose. Most active at dawn and dusk, they feed on plants found primarily in wetlands. If you do spot a moose, give it generous clearance, as they can be unpredictably aggressive. Just south of town, the trail traverses the protected Salmon Brook Bog Area, home to hundreds of species of flora and fauna.

The southern section of the BAT runs north of Houlton, ending just shy of Presque Isle in the tiny town of Phair, where the railroad siding once connected to a company potato house. To continue north to Presque Isle, you'll need to follow an ATV trail.

DIRECTIONS

To reach the trailhead off US Hwy. 1 in Caribou, where food, lodging, and trail information are available, take State Route 89 east for 0.4 mile and turn left at the sign for trailhead parking.

Contact: Caribou Parks & Recreation
55 Bennett Drive
Caribou, ME 04736
(207) 493-4224
www.caribourec.org

Calais Waterfront Walkway

FINISH

Franklin St

South St

Palmer Ln

Main St

Hill St

Eaton St

Barker St

Elm St

Swan St

Tyler St

Downes St

Temperance St

Winter St

Lafayette St

Park St

Washington St

Germain St

Church St

Spring St

Sawyer St

Calais

Pikes Park

P

Visitor Center

START

Lowell St

Calais Ave

Lincoln St

Main St

Buick St

Monroe St

1

Whitney St

High St

McLean St

River St

Union St

Carver St

North St

Garfield St

Price St

Chandler St

Pleasant St

Pool St

St Croix River

St Croix River

Todd St

FINISH

N

0   0.1   0.2   0.3   0.4 Mile

rails·to·trails
conservancy

Calais Waterfront Walkway

At the heart of town, the 1.4-mile Calais Waterfront Walkway follows the route of the former Maine Central Line, though the original bed dates to the Calais Railway, chartered in 1832—the first charter issued by the state of Maine. Crews have transformed the right-of-way into a promenade that skirts the St. Croix River from South Street to Todd Street.

The trailhead is at Pikes Park, the trail midpoint. Whether you head east or west, you're guaranteed scenic vistas. Pause en route to peruse interpretive exhibits at the Downeast Maine Heritage Center or watch bald eagles scan the water from perches just feet from the trail. The city hopes to expand the walkway to 3 miles and link it to other trails in the St. Croix Valley.

On the opposite shore is St. Stephen, New Brunswick, Canada, which is developing its own system of waterfront parks and trails. If you want to check it out, it's within easy walking distance. The Waterfront Walkway passes within a hundred yards of the international bridge.

Location
Washington County

Endpoints
South Street to
Todd Street

Mileage
1.4

Roughness Index
2

Surface
Gravel

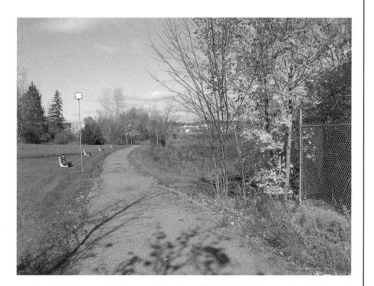

The Calais Waterfront Walkway provides views of the St. Croix River along its 1.4-mile path.

DIRECTIONS

To reach the trailhead at Pikes Park, take State Route 9 east to its junction with US Hwy. 1, turn right, and follow signs to downtown Calais. The road becomes North Street, and the park is on the waterfront.

Contact: City of Calais
PO Box 413
Calais, ME 04619
(207) 454-2521
www.calaismaine.govoffice.com

Eastern Promenade Trail

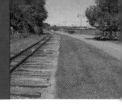

Portland is Maine's largest city, and the 2.1-mile Eastern Promenade Trail along Casco Bay offers an ideal introduction to this coastal town and its trail network.

The "East Prom" begins in Old Port, a charming waterfront district with cobblestone streets and working piers. A massive brick foundry that once turned out steam engines now houses the trailside Maine Narrow Gauge Railroad Company & Museum. Outside, cheerfully restored narrow gauge train cars—including a bright red Ocean Spray boxcar—stand ready for service. For a nostalgic lark, take an out-and-back excursion on the slender railcars (narrow gauge rails stand just 2 feet apart). You'll skirt most of the trail's route.

Take the side path up to Fort Allen Park to search for a battleship cannon, or stay on the trail and look southeast to spot Fort Gorges, which was armed and active during the Civil and Spanish-American wars. You'll reach the trail midpoint at East End Beach, where all-weather kayakers launch into the surf.

From here, eponymous Eastern Promenade Park flanks the trail for a mile. Near the north end of the park,

Location
Cumberland County

Endpoints
Old Port to Back Cove Loop Trail, Portland

Mileage
2.1

Roughness Index
1

Surface
Asphalt

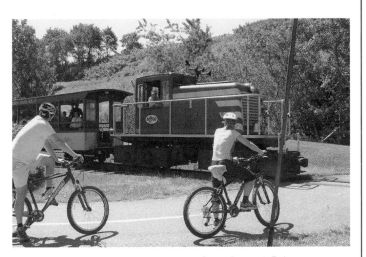

An out-and-back excursion train runs along the Eastern Promenade Trail.

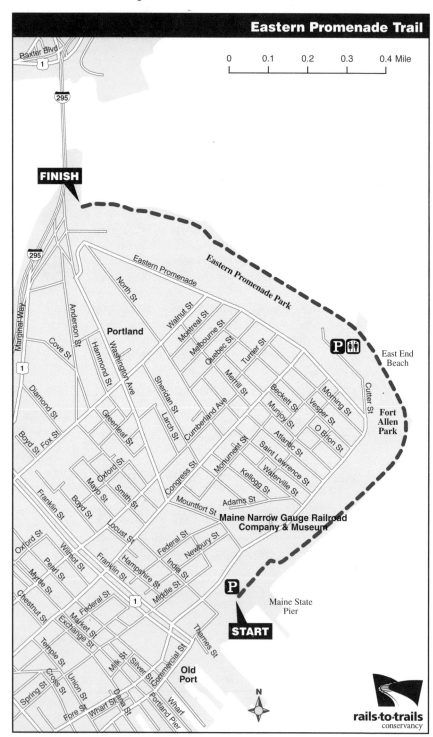

Eastern Promenade Trail

0   0.1   0.2   0.3   0.4 Mile

Baxter Blvd

1

295

FINISH

295

Marginal Way

Eastern Promenade

Eastern Promenade Park

North St

Anderson St

Cove St

1

Diamond St

Hammond St

Washington Ave

Portland

Walnut St

Montreal St

Melbourne St

Quebec St

Turner St

P 🚻

East End Beach

Boyd St   Fox St

Greenleaf St

Sheridan St

Larch St

Cumberland Ave

Merrill St

Beckett St

Munjoy St

O Brion St

Vesper St

Morning St

Cutter St

Fort Allen Park

Oxford St

Mayo St

Smith St

Boyd St

Congress St

Monument St

Saint Lawrence St

Atlantic St

Waterville St

Kellogg St

Franklin St

Locust St

Mountfort St

Adams St

Maine Narrow Gauge Railroad Company & Museum

Oxford St

Wilmot St

Pearl St

Myrtle St

Franklin St

Federal St

Hampshire St

India St

Middle St

Federal St

Newbury St

P

Maine State Pier

START

Chestnut St

Federal St

Market St

Exchange St

Milk St

Silver St

Commercial St

Thames St

Temple St

Cross St

Union St

Wharf St

Dana St

Portland Pier

Wharf

Old Port

Spring St

Fore St

N

rails·to·trails
conservancy

the rail-trail detours from the rail corridor up a short hill. From its rise, scan the bay for the remains of an old swing bridge that extends a third of a mile over the water. This majestic span was once part of the Grand Trunk Railway between Quebec and Maine.

At the crest of the hill, just past the city's water-treatment plant and a colorful mural, the rail-trail nears its end. From here, you can backtrack to Old Port or continue along the Back Cove Loop Trail.

DIRECTIONS

To reach the India Street trailhead, take Interstate 295 to the Franklin Avenue exit and follow it until it dead-ends at Commercial Street in Old Port. Turn left and drive to the end of the street. The trailhead is at the intersection of Commercial and India.

Parking and restrooms are available at the East End Beach boat launch, at the end of Cutter Street along the East Prom.

Contact: Portland Trails
305 Commercial Street
Portland, ME 04101
(207) 775-2411

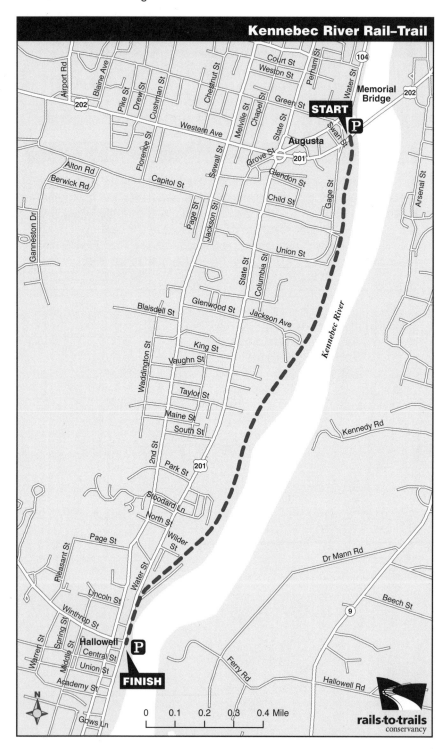

Kennebec River Rail-Trail

A stunning gateway to Maine's capital city, the Kennebec River Rail-Trail follows the railroad right-of-way that once connected Portland to Augusta. The trail parallels the inactive railroad tracks, which have been maintained in the hope they will one day be used again. Granite quarter-mile markers mimic the original larger markers the railroad once used.

The trail also follows the 120-mile Kennebec River, a historic waterway named by the Abnaki Indians and meaning "long, quiet waters." Once extremely polluted, the river is now a thriving habitat for fish and wildlife, largely due to clean water laws and removal of the Edwards Dam, built in Augusta back in 1837. Atlantic salmon, striped bass, and American shad, as well as alewife, blueback herring, and rainbow smelt, visit the Kennebec, which also shelters one of the few extant breeding populations of the rare Atlantic sturgeon. Don't be surprised if you spot a bald eagle soaring the river in hopes of a good catch.

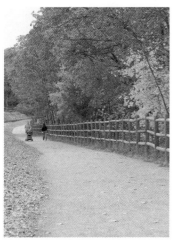

The Kennebec River Rail-Trail closely follows its namesake river for 2 miles from Augusta to Hallowell.

The trail begins beneath Augusta's Memorial Bridge, where you'll find parking and a trailhead information kiosk. Heading south along this asphalt-paved stretch, you'll soon leave the capital city's hustle and bustle behind. The picturesque Kennebec flows to your left, while a high slope on the right shields you from the nearby capitol complex. At about the half-mile marker, look across the river to the Kennebec Arsenal, whose massive stone buildings are to be developed and repurposed into commercial and residential housing units.

Location
Kennebec County

Endpoints
Augusta to Hallowell

Mileage
2

Roughness Index
1

Surface
Asphalt, crushed stone

Near the 1-mile marker, a side path leads down to the trail from the State Capitol complex. Constructed of native granite, the building's portico and front facade, with a towering arcade, is the work of noted American architect Charles Bulfinch.

Between the 1.5- and 1.75-mile markers, the trail curves to the right. Here, the surface changes from asphalt to firmly packed stone dust. Note the massive stone blocks that form a retaining wall farther south on the inland side of the corridor. As a white church steeple comes into view, the trail diverges from the rail corridor and enters the town of Hallowell, where you'll find a variety of shops and eateries.

Work is underway to complete the final 3-mile section of trail from Hallowell to Farmingdale, where it will connect with an existing milelong segment to Gardiner.

DIRECTIONS

To reach the Augusta trailhead, take Interstate 95 to Exit 30B and head east on State Route 202. Follow 202 to the traffic circle and take State Route 201 south. At the second set of lights, turn left, and then turn right into the trailhead parking lot.

Contact: Friends of the Kennebec River Rail-Trail
PO Box 2195
Augusta, ME 04338
www.krrt.org

Kennebec Valley Trail

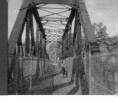

The quiet Kennebec Valley Trail (a.k.a. Anson to Bingham Trail) boasts surprising claims to fame: The 14.6-mile trail traces the river and Indian path taken in 1775 by Benedict Arnold, on orders from General George Washington, to capture Quebec from the British; it also follows a historic narrow gauge logging railroad and, at one point, is bisected by the 45th parallel.

The surface is largely packed dirt and crushed stone. Despite intermittent rolling dips from ATV use on the sandy stretches, the trail nevertheless delivers a good mountain bike ride.

While the trail has only been fully developed from south of Solon to Bingham, additional undeveloped (read: less manicured) trail miles stretch north from the North Anson cemetery, nearly doubling the overall length. The line originated as a narrow gauge logging railroad, then hauled freight and passengers up around Moosehead Lake, Maine's largest.

North of Solon, tremendous views of the Kennebec River compensate for occasional rough going on the trail. The river is so wide in places, you may have to remind yourself you're traveling alongside a mighty river

Location
Somerset County

Endpoints
North Anson to Bingham

Mileage
14.6

Roughness Index
3

Surface
Crushed stone, dirt, sand

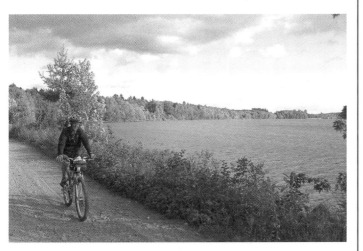

The Kennebec Valley Trail offers stunning views across the Kennebec River.

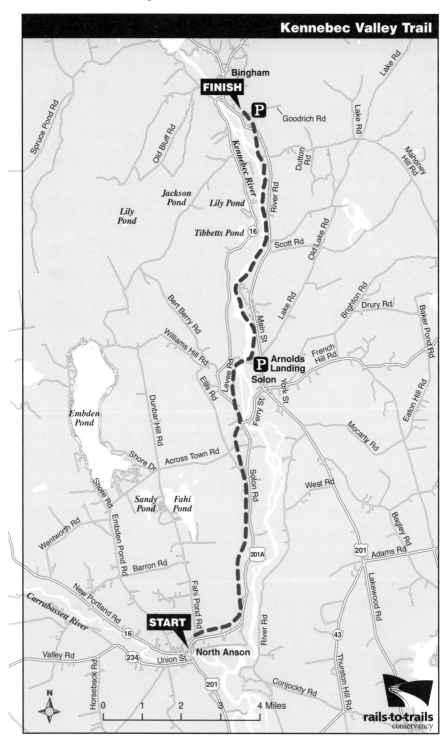

Kennebec Valley Trail

Bingham
FINISH
P
Goodrich Rd
Lake Rd
Spruce Pond Rd
Old Bluff Rd
Kennebec River
Jackson Pond
Lily Pond
Lily Pond
Tibbetts Pond 16
Scott Rd
River Rd
Dutton Rd
Mahoney Hill Rd
Old Lake Rd
Bert Berry Rd
Lake Rd
Main St
Brighton Rd
Drury Rd
Baker Pond Rd
Williams Hill Rd
Ellis Rd
Levee Rd
P Arnolds Landing
Solon
French Hill Rd
York St
Ferry St
Eaton Hill Rd
Dunbar Hill Rd
Embden Pond
Shore Dr
Across Town Rd
Mccarty Rd
West Rd
Solon Rd
Bagley Rd
Shore Rd
Sandy Pond
Fahi Pond
Wentworth Rd
Embden Pond Rd
Barron Rd
201A
201
Adams Rd
Lakewood Rd
New Portland Rd
Fahi Pond Rd
START
16
Carrabassett River
Valley Rd
234
Union St
North Anson
River Rd
43
Thurston Hill Rd
201
Conjockty Rd
Horseback Rd

N

0   1   2   3   4 Miles

rails·to·trails
conservancy

and not one of Maine's beautiful lakes. Listen for the cry of loons, especially around dusk; if you're really lucky, you may even spot one up close.

At an electrical generating station near Arnolds Landing (north of Solon), the trail spans a former railroad bridge across the Kennebec. North of the landing, the trail runs within feet of the river for long expanses. Unless you're carrying a GPS receiver, you won't be aware when you cross the 45th parallel—the theoretical midpoint between the equator and the North Pole. You'll eventually emerge at the Bingham trailhead on Goodrich Road.

DIRECTIONS

To reach the North Anson trailhead, take US Hwy. 201A to town and turn west on Fahi Pond Road. The trail starts on the right just before the cemetery.

To reach the Bingham trailhead, take US Hwy. 201 south through town and turn left on Goodrich Road. The parking lot is on the left, with trail access on the right.

Contact: Maine Department of Conservation
Bureau of Parks & Lands
22 State House Station
18 Elkins Lane (AMHI Campus)
Augusta, ME 04333
(207) 287-4957
www.state.me.us/doc/parks

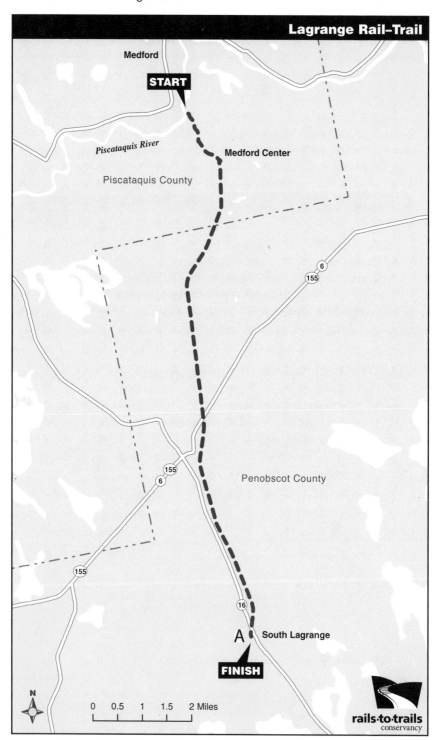

Lagrange Rail–Trail

Medford

START

Piscataquis River

Medford Center

Piscataquis County

6
155

Penobscot County

155
6

155

16

A South Lagrange

FINISH

N

0   0.5   1   1.5   2 Miles

rails·to·trails
conservancy

Lagrange Rail-Trail

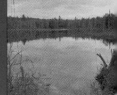

The Piscataquis River bisects the tiny village of Medford (population 231). The north bank is known as Medford; the south bank is Medford Center. Before the Bangor & Aroostook Railroad opened a 600-foot-long, 60-foot-high trestle across the river in 1907, a ferry hauled supplies, produce, and people across the water. Eventually, ferry service ceased, and the freight line provided the only river crossing in the area. Citizens in Medford Center wanting to conduct municipal business were forced to travel a 40-mile route. When the railroad abandoned the line, more daring townspeople resorted to crossing the open ties of the trestle on foot and by car.

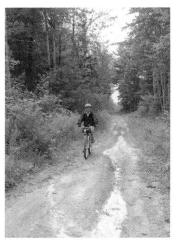

This rough rail-trail features wildlife and a 600-foot-long resurfaced railroad.

As crews prepared to remove the trestle, the town stepped in to purchase and retrofit it. The newly resurfaced bridge opened in 1981, and today cars, pedestrians, bicycles, ATVs, and snowmobiles share the span. This bridge kicks off your trip on the 11-mile Lagrange Rail-Trail (a.k.a. Lagrange Right-of-Way).

The first few miles south of the river are rough, and even a light rain can fill the gullies, making it difficult to navigate. Cyclists must use a mountain bike. Less than a mile from the bridge, the trail threads through quaint Medford Center, whose few buildings cluster around a restored barn that serves as the town hall. Just past an old church, the trail crosses the paved road and then widens, becoming much more navigable.

Much of the trail is shaded by tree canopy, interspersed with ponds that reflect the vast Maine sky. The

Location
Piscataquis and Penobscot counties

Endpoints
Medford to South Lagrange

Mileage
11

Roughness Index
3

Surface
Crushed stone, dirt

trail passes a particularly beautiful pond about midway between Medford Center and Lagrange. These ponds and bogs are wildlife magnets and open for fishing access. Watch closely for moose tracks, as moose use the trail to move from bog to bog. Should you encounter a moose, use extreme caution, as they can be unpredictably aggressive.

DIRECTIONS

To access the trail from Medford, cross the trestle and drive 0.3 mile along an unsigned dirt road till it bends to the left. Park along the shoulder.

Contact: Lagrange & Alton Snowmobile Club
3346 Bennoch Road
Alton, ME 04468
(207) 394-2981

Mountain Division Trail

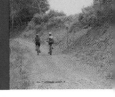

Named for the railroad line it parallels, the Mountain Division Trail provides a gently rolling excursion in the rural Sebago Lake Watershed Area, northwest of Portland. The trail extends 4.8 miles from Standish to Windham. Maine's Department of Transportation owns the onward section between South Windham and Fryeburg and has yet to develop it. Trail advocates hope the entire route will someday connect with Portland's well-developed trail network.

Start from the western trailhead at Johnson Field in Standish. Pause at the trailhead kiosk to fill out a registration form for use of the parkland within the watershed. From the large parking area, you'll follow a dirt road trafficked in summer by local YMCA campers. The road undulates past stands of mixed conifer and deciduous trees for about a half mile before reaching the trail.

Technically, the Mountain Division Trail is a rail-with-trail (see more on rails-with-trails on page 2), although the rail is no longer active. Narrow in places with steep embankments, the roller-coaster trail sometimes runs level with the tracks and sometimes dips below. The

Location
Cumberland County

Endpoints
Standish to Windham

Mileage
4.8

Roughness Index
2.5

Surface
Crushed stone, dirt

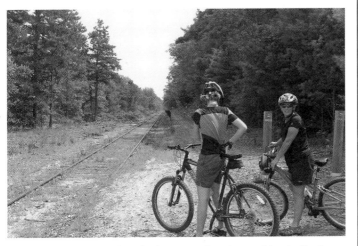

Though no trains run on the tracks, the presence of an adjacent rail line classifies the Mountain Division Trail as a rail-with-trail.

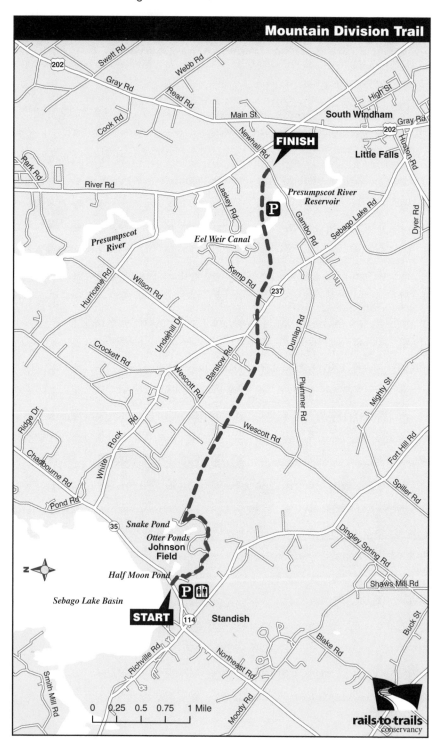

Mountain Division Trail

soothing aroma of balsam fir permeates the air, especially near the Presumpscot River.

DIRECTIONS

To reach the trailhead at Johnson Field in Standish, take State Route 35 to its intersection with State Route 114. The parking area is on 35, a quarter mile east of the intersection.
You'll find limited roadside parking in Windham.

Contact: Mountain Division Alliance
PO Box 532
Fryeburg, ME 04037
(207) 935-4283
www.mountaindivisiontrail.org

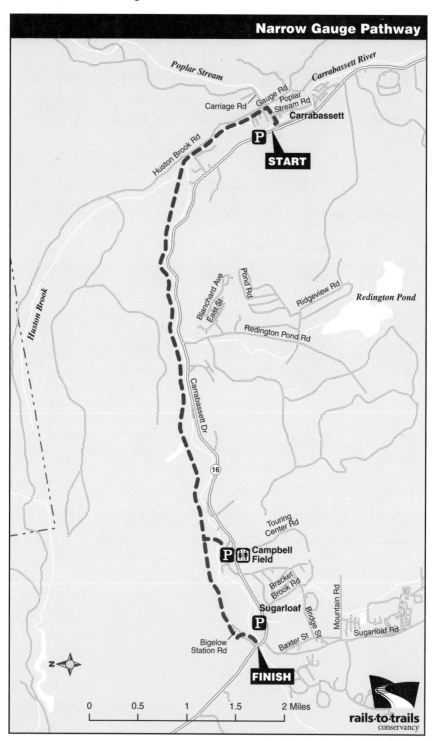

Narrow Gauge Pathway

Poplar Stream

Carrabassett River

Carriage Rd

Gauge Rd

Poplar Stream Rd

Carrabassett

Huston Brook Rd

P

START

Blanchard Ave

Pond Rd

East St

Ridgeview Rd

Redington Pond

Redington Pond Rd

Huston Brook

Carrabassett Dr

16

Touring Center Rd

P **Campbell Field**

Bracket Brook Rd

Mountain Rd

Sugarloaf

P

Bridge St

Sugarloaf Rd

Bigelow Station Rd

Baxter St

N

FINISH

| 0 | 0.5 | 1 | 1.5 | 2 Miles |

rails·to·trails
conservancy

Narrow Gauge Pathway

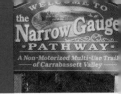

The Narrow Gauge Pathway (a.k.a. Carrabassett River Trail) is a stunningly beautiful 6.6-mile trail along the banks of the Carrabassett River. Its firm, crushed-stone surface is suitable for mountain bike or hybrid tires. The pathway is also popular among hikers and cross-country skiers.

For a solid workout on a gradual but steady uphill climb, start from the Carrabassett town office trailhead. The return trip from the entrance to Sugarloaf USA ski resort is downhill all the way and a joy to ride.

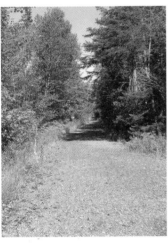

This rural trail takes its names from the narrow gauge rail car that once ran on the corridor.

The trail is named for a 2-foot-wide narrow gauge line operated by the Kingfield & Dead River Railroad around the turn of the century. Popular throughout Maine, narrow gauge railways were ideal for rough terrain. As logging was the primary industry, most of Sugarloaf's trails echo logging terms.

Picnic tables dot the trail, and in summer you'll find spots to cool your feet or take a dip in the river. Trailside wildflowers bloom in profusion from early spring through fall, while birch, aspen, and maples offer splashes of spectacular color during the fall foliage season.

Crossing a 400-foot boardwalk over a beaver flowage, you'll reach the Campbell Field trailhead, about 5 miles along the pathway. A great spot to watch for the busy dam builders, the trailhead provides a comfort station, including a restroom and small parking lot.

Location
Franklin County

Endpoints
Carrabassett to Sugarloaf USA

Mileage
6.6

Roughness Index
3

Surface
Crushed stone, dirt

DIRECTIONS

To reach the trailhead in Carrabassett, drive north on State Route 27, turn right on Carriage Road, and cross the bridge. Park at the municipal lot on the left. The signed trailhead is on the road.

To reach the Sugarloaf USA trailhead, head north on Route 27 toward the ski resort. Pass the main entrance on your left and continue 100 feet across a concrete bridge. The trailhead will be on your right. Parking is available in the large lot at the Antigravity Center, just left of the main entrance to Sugarloaf.

Contact: Town of Carrabassett Valley
1001 Carriage Road
Carrabassett Valley, ME 04947
(207) 235-2645
www.carrabassettvalley.org

Newport–Dover-Foxcroft Rail-Trail

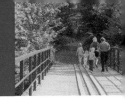

In central Maine, the Newport–Dover-Foxcroft Rail-Trail (a.k.a. Moosehead Trail) links five towns, two rivers, three lakes, and a range of pristine landscapes. Extending from State Route 7 in Newport to its northern terminus near Fairview Street in Dover-Foxcroft, the corridor is used by hikers, bicyclists, cross-country skiers, dogsledders, equestrians, snowmobilers, and ATV users. An alternative route between the towns of Newport, Corinna, Dexter, Sangerville, and Dover-Foxcroft, the trail also links to the central Maine Interconnected Trail System.

Despite busy weekends, the trail affords a very pleasant mountain bike trek, with plenty of side trips and places to stop for provisions. In summer, watch for the many humps and dips in the soft surface, which puddle after excessive rains. The trail borders lakes and streams and traverses farmland, woodland, and wetland areas.

In Newport, the trail briefly skirts the shore of Sebasticook Lake and its charming lakeside residences. Farther along, where the trail crosses State Route 7/11 in Corinna, an intriguing antique shop, general store, and

Location
Penobscot and Piscataquis counties

Endpoints
Newport to Dover-Foxcroft

Mileage
26.5

Roughness Index
3

Surface
Crushed stone, dirt, sand

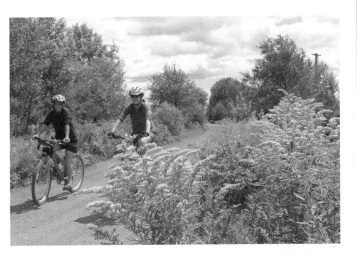

The Newport–Dover-Foxcroft Rail-Trail connects five towns and is part of Maine's Interconnected Trail System.

Newport–Dover–Foxcroft Rail-Trail

café provide local color and a relaxing diversion. Rejoining the trail, you'll glimpse the east branch of the Sebasticook River.

The town of Dexter (once the home of Dexter shoes) offers a grocery and sandwich shop, as well as a trail link to Lake Wassookeag. Summer wildflowers line the trail just north of town.

DIRECTIONS

To reach the Newport trailhead, take Interstate 95 to State Route 7 north. Trailhead parking is on the right side of Route 7, just north of the town center.

The Dover-Foxcroft trailhead is near the junction of state routes 7, 15, and 6. From the junction, travel west on 6 just over a mile. Trailhead parking is on the right, by Irving's Gas Station.

Contact: Maine Department of Conservation
Bureau of Parks & Lands
22 State House Station
18 Elkins Lane (AMHI Campus)
Augusta, ME 04333
(207) 287-5574
www.state.me.us/doc/parks

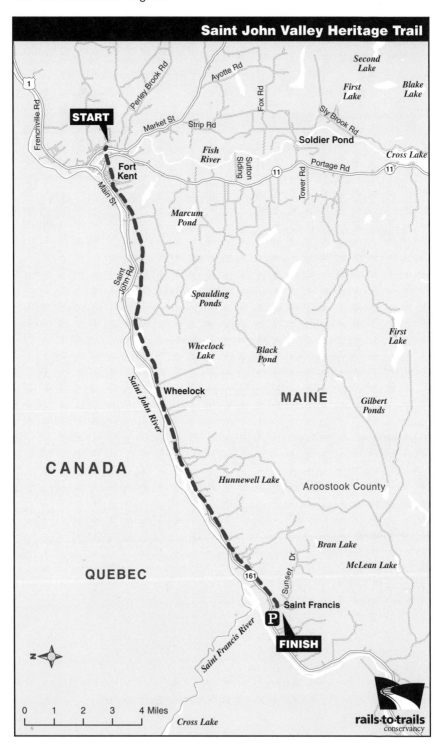

Saint John Valley Heritage Trail

Second Lake

First Lake

Blake Lake

Perley Brook Rd

Ayotte Rd

Fox Rd

1

Frenchville Rd

START

Market St

Strip Rd

Sly Brook Rd

Soldier Pond

Cross Lake

Fort Kent

Main St

Fish River

Sutton Siding

11

Tower Rd

Portage Rd

11

Saint John Rd

Marcum Pond

Spaulding Ponds

First Lake

Wheelock Lake

Black Pond

Saint John River

Wheelock

MAINE

Gilbert Ponds

CANADA

Hunnewell Lake

Aroostook County

Bran Lake

QUEBEC

McLean Lake

161

Sunset Dr

Saint Francis

P

FINISH

Saint Francis River

N

0   1   2   3   4 Miles

Cross Lake

rails·to·trails
conservancy

Saint John Valley Heritage Trail

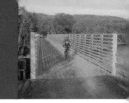

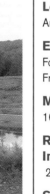

The Saint John Valley Heritage Trail traces 16.9 miles of the former Fish River Railroad corridor, which was taken over by the Bangor & Aroostook Railroad, a line that transported goods and passengers across northern Maine. Skirting the Saint John River, the well-maintained, crushed-stone trail offers views of the forests, farmlands, and wetlands on the Canadian side of the river.

Start your trail exploration in the historic town of Fort Kent. The wooden blockhouse is the only remnant of the Aroostook War of 1838–1839, a border dispute between Maine and New Brunswick that was settled without any actual fighting. The fort is on Blockhouse Road, at the confluence of the Fish and Saint John rivers.

Your first stop should be the restored 1902 train station, which served as the Fish River Railroad terminus. Now owned by the Fort Kent Historical Society, it houses a museum devoted to the railroad.

Back on the trail, you'll soon cross a pedestrian bridge over the Fish River. As the trail continues through Fort Kent, watch for road crossings and spurs that lead to restaurants, service stations, and other businesses.

Location
Aroostook County

Endpoints
Fort Kent to Saint Francis

Mileage
16.9

Roughness Index
2

Surface
Crushed stone

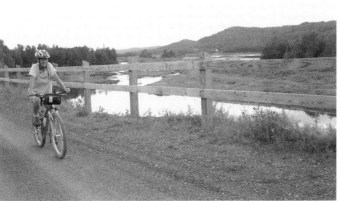

The Saint John Valley Heritage Trail traces the Saint John River between Canada and the US.

Beyond town, the trail passes through forests and wetlands along the banks of the Saint John.

Although the trail parallels State Route 161 for several miles, the mixed forest remains quiet and serene. In the town of Wheelock, the trail crosses to the north side of 161. This section offers the best views of villages and farms in New Brunswick. When you reach the town of Saint John, the trail again crosses Route 161, passing behind homes and shops. Exercise caution, as this is a busy road.

Nearing the trail's end in Saint Francis, you'll pass a railroad turntable recently restored by Fort Kent High School students, who also built a path leading into town. The trail soon ends at a large parking lot and trailhead.

DIRECTIONS

The Fort Kent trailhead is behind the Citgo station on Market Street, while State Route 161 is lined with access points.

To reach the Saint Francis trailhead, take Route 161 to Sunset Drive. Parking is on the left, just past the church.

Contact: Fort Kent Office of Economic Development
416 West Main Street
Fort Kent, ME 04743
(207) 834-3136
www.fortkent.org

Sipayik Trail

On the Pleasant Point Reservation abutting coastal New Brunswick, this paved rail-trail was built to keep Passamaquoddy youngsters off busy Route 190, which connects Pleasant Point with Eastport and runs through the middle of the reservation.

The 1.7-mile trail meanders through the woods, with the tidal Little River and Atlantic Ocean on one side and a grassy marsh on the other. Over much of its course, the Sipayik overlooks a spectacular coastline, highlighted by views of nearby Deer Island. Beach access is permitted from the trail.

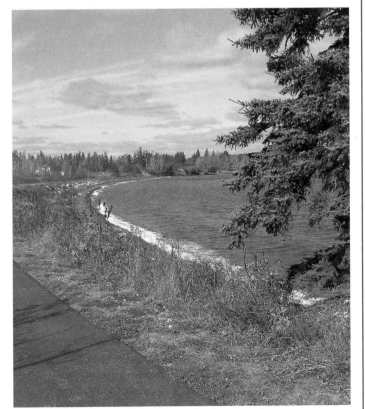

The Sipayik Trail provides a walk- and bike-able connection between the Pleasant Point Reservation and local businesses, schools, and recreation areas.

Location
Washington County

Endpoints
Within the Pleasant Point Indian Reservation

Mileage
1.7

Roughness Index
1

Surface
Asphalt

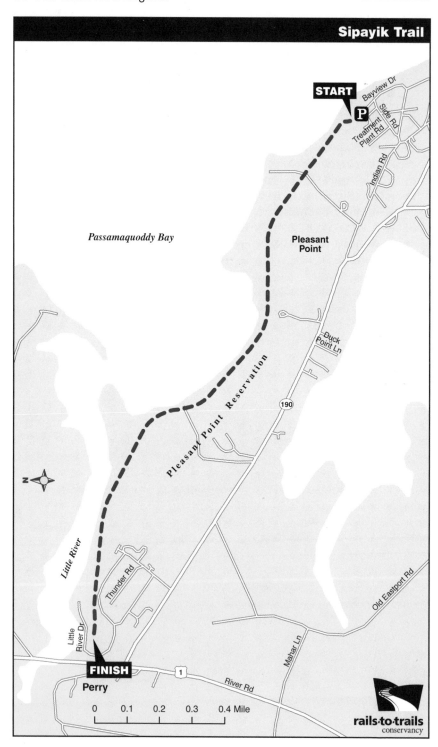

Sipayik Trail

START

P

Bayview Dr

Side Rd

Treatment
Plant Rd

Indian Rd

Passamaquoddy Bay

Pleasant
Point

Duck
Point Ln

190

Pleasant Point Reservation

Little River

Thunder Rd

Old Eastport Rd

N

Little
River Dr

FINISH

Perry

1

River Rd

Mahar Ln

0   0.1   0.2   0.3   0.4 Mile

rails·to·trails
conservancy

DIRECTIONS

To access the Sipayik Trail, take US Hwy. 1 to State Route 190 east. In Pleasant Point, turn left on Indian Road, left on Middle Road, and left again on Side Road. At the bottom of the hill, follow Treatment Plant Road to trail parking at road's end.

Contact: Passamaquoddy Tribe at Pleasant Point
PO Box 343
Route 190
Perry, ME 04667
(207) 853-2600
www.wabanaki.com/index.html

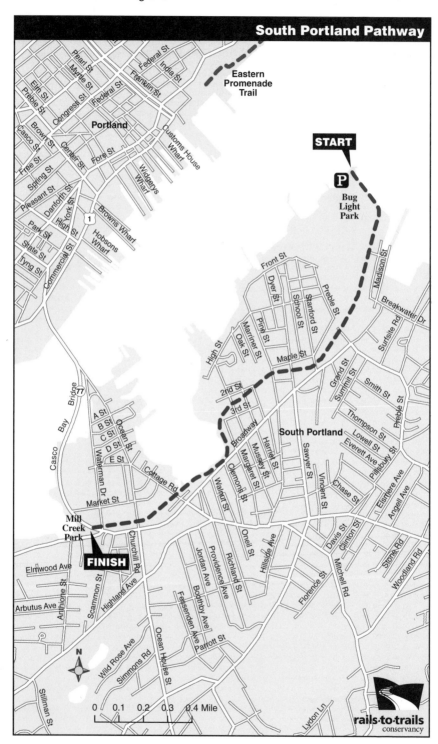

South Portland Pathway

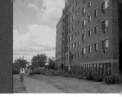

An exemplary urban transportation corridor, the 5.7-mile South Portland Parkway (2.1 miles of which are rail-trail) makes an excellent starting point for a bike tour of Portland. The trailhead at Bug Light Park offers easy access and plenty of free parking, and it connects to Portland's extensive network of walking and bicycling trails.

Small bollards and yellow street signs mark the route and indicate the distance to other parts of town. The pathway—also known as the South Portland Greenbelt—links residential areas, schools (both elementary and collegiate), marinas, parks, rec centers, assisted-living facilities, and retail hubs.

Named for the watchful lighthouse at the tip of the breakwater, Bug Light Park was once home to the Portland Shipyard, which produced hundreds of Liberty Ships, the workhorses of the US Navy during World War II. The park opened in 1989, thanks to public contributions and support from the South Portland–Cape Elizabeth Rotary Club. Here, you can watch for passing sailboats, tankers off-loading oil bound for Montreal, and arriving ferries from New Brunswick and Nova Scotia.

Location
Cumberland County

Endpoints
Bug Light Park to Mill Creek Park

Mileage
2.1

Roughness Index
1

Surface
Asphalt

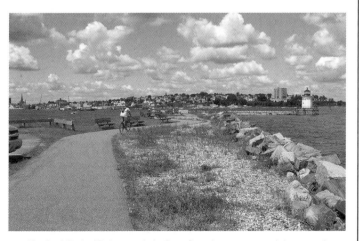

The South Portland Pathway overlooks Casco Bay, where you can watch ferries travel to and from New Brunswick and Nova Scotia.

Marking the end of the rail-trail portion is the Casco Bay Bridge, which curls across the Fore River, connecting the neighborhoods of South Portland with downtown's sophisticated shops and eateries. A walkway spans the bridge, affording views of the bay and city skyline.

DIRECTIONS

To reach Bug Light Park from Portland, take Interstate 295 to Exit 6A and follow State Route 77 across the Casco Bay Bridge. Continue straight (don't follow Route 77) on Broadway to the T-junction, turn left on Breakwater Drive, then right on Madison Street. Follow signs for the lighthouse to the parking lot.

Contact: Portland Trails
305 Commercial Street
Portland, ME 04101
(207) 775-2411

Whistle Stop Rail-Trail

The Whistle Stop is a textbook example of how diverse groups can work together to maintain and promote a trail. Developed as a route for snowmobilers and off-roaders, the route also appeals to hikers and mountain bikers. It's no wonder. The 13-mile corridor spans the range of environments Maine's Western Mountain region has to offer. Never far from small community centers, the trail meanders through residential areas, then plunges back into wetland wilderness and beaver habitat. The trail's sandy, sometimes rutted surface and trailside pine and mixed deciduous forest demand your attention.

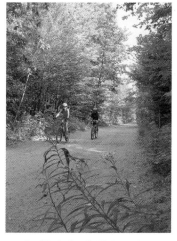

The Whistle Stop Rail-Trail cuts through wilderness areas in between stops in small towns built around the white granite industry.

While the trail is accessible from numerous points in Jay, Wilton, and Farmington, Farmington offers the best trailhead parking. Just south of the trailhead is another inviting feature—a warming hut that centers on a wood-burning stove stocked with a ready supply of split wood. Sponsored by Franklin Memorial Hospital, the yurt also offers instructional signs for fitness exercises. Signs direct trail users down a quarter-mile side trail to the health center's restrooms and café.

Farther along the Whistle Stop, you'll cross several bridges redecked by area snowmobile and ATV clubs. These span scenic Sevenmile Stream, part of the massive Androscoggin watershed.

North of Jay, a large, granite-block embankment marks the site of the old North Jay Quarry. The Maine and New Hampshire Granite Corporation operated along the railbed from 1886 until the early 1900s. Crews

Location
Franklin County

Endpoints
Farmington to Jay

Mileage
13

Roughness Index
3

Surface
Crushed stone, dirt, sand

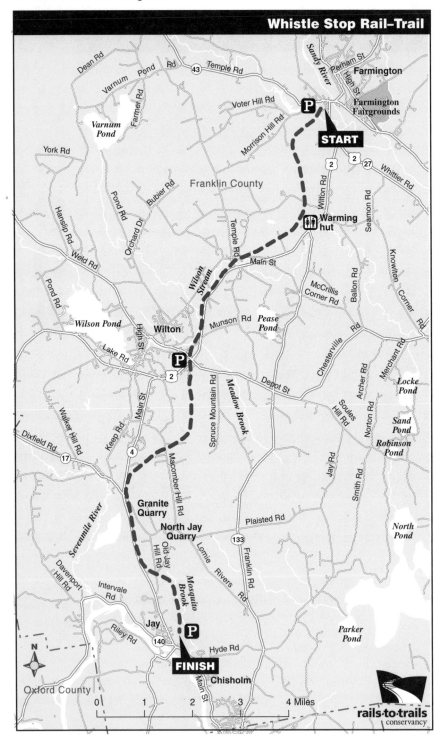

Whistle Stop Rail–Trail

would cut and haul large blocks of white granite along a rail siding to a cutting shed, where the blocks were further shaped and sculpted for use in buildings across the country. Interpretive signs tell the story and include historical photographs of the quarry. A mile shy of the trail's end in Jay, you'll reach a large dirt parking lot at the intersection with Maine Interconnected Trail System 84.

DIRECTIONS

To reach the Farmington trailhead, head into town on US Hwy. 2 and take Bridge Street to the four-way stop. Turn left here on Oaks Street, then turn right on Farmer Lane to the trailhead parking area.

Trailhead parking in Jay lies just off the southeast side of State Route 4/17.

Contact: Maine Department of Conservation
Bureau of Parks & Lands
22 State House Station
18 Elkins Lane (AMHI Campus)
Augusta, ME 04333
(207) 287-4958
www.state.me.us/doc/parks

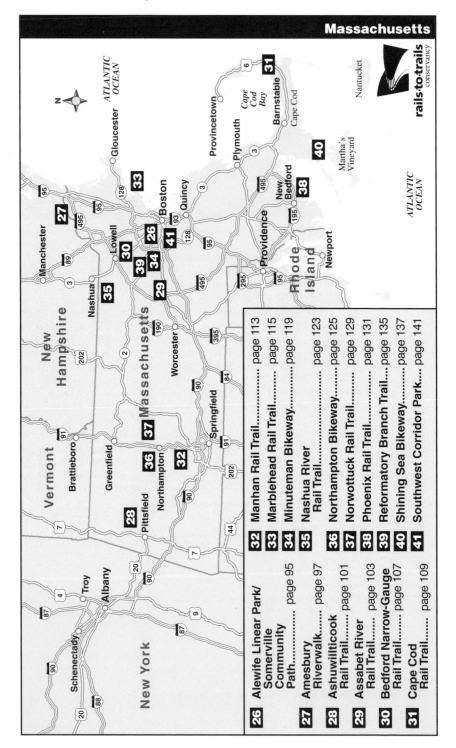

rails·to·trails
conservancy

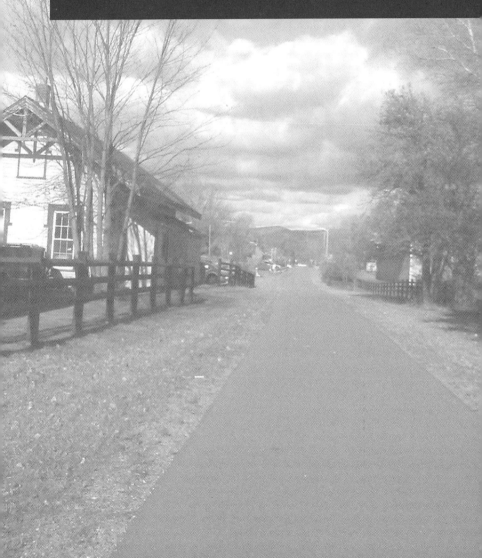

Massachusetts

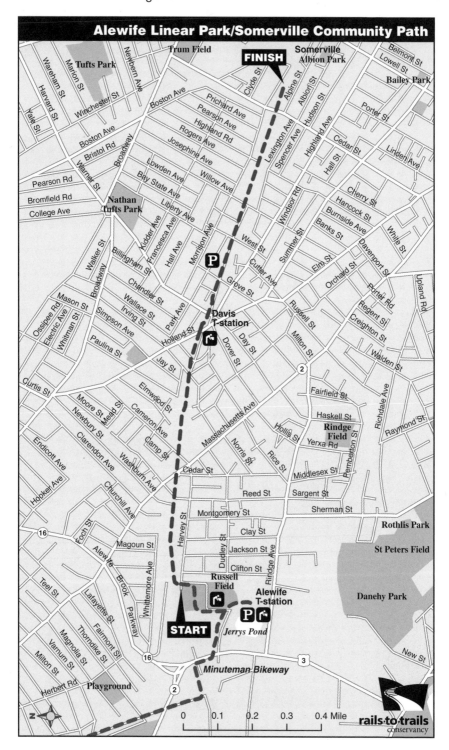

Alewife Linear Park/Somerville Community Path

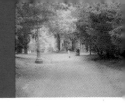

Alewife Linear Park is a beautiful paved trail stretching 2 miles east from the Alewife T-station in Cambridge to Cedar Street in Somerville. The park came about after the Massachusetts Bay Transportation Authority put its Red Line underground; between the Alewife and Davis T-stations, the subway runs directly beneath the trail. The trail's urban/suburban locale and its direct link to the 11-mile Minuteman Bikeway (see page 119) makes this a busy commuter and recreation corridor. Note that while dogs are not permitted on the trail, local residents often break this rule. Watch where you step.

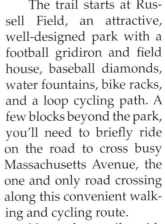

In the northwest suburbs of Boston, several rail-trails link communities with public transportation.

The trail starts at Russell Field, an attractive, well-designed park with a football gridiron and field house, baseball diamonds, water fountains, bike racks, and a loop cycling path. A few blocks beyond the park, you'll need to briefly ride on the road to cross busy Massachusetts Avenue, the one and only road crossing along this convenient walking and cycling route.

Near the trail midpoint, a tree-lined brick path leads directly to the Davis T-station. The trail here is sometimes referred to as the Somerville Community Path. Several wind-activated structures on brick-and-steel pillars depict scenes of historical Somerville. Cyclists may use any of the numerous bike racks and, outside of rush hour, you may choose to take your bike on the train for a further exploration of metro Boston.

Or continue past the station, through the hip Davis Square neighborhood and back onto the Alewife Linear

Location
Middlesex County

Endpoints
Alewife T-station in Cambridge to Cedar Street in Somerville

Mileage
2

Roughness Index
1

Surface
Asphalt

Park/Somerville Community Path for almost another mile toward downtown Somerville. Along the way, you'll pass a couple of parks, including one with a playground. Nearing trail's end, the surface changes to woodchips for about 100 feet before reaching the tracks and ties of the old railroad. One day, this trail may extend to the end of the line in Somerville, but until then, it is advised that you stop at the official trail end.

DIRECTIONS

By subway, take the Red Line to Alewife or Davis Square. Bicycles are permitted on subways during off-peak hours on weekdays or all day on weekends. To reach the Alewife T-station—and trail parking—take Interstate 95 to Exit 29A and head east on the Concord Turnpike/State Route 2 toward Arlington and Cambridge. At the end of the turnpike, bear right on Alewife Brook Parkway, then turn right on Cambridge Park Drive. The station is on the right, and the trailhead is behind the parking garage. For more information, visit www.mbta.com.

Contact: City of Somerville
93 Highland Avenue
Somerville, MA 02143
(617) 625-6600

Amesbury Riverwalk

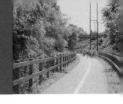

A lovely, albeit short rail-trail in northeastern Massachusetts, the 1.3-mile Amesbury Riverwalk (a.k.a. Powwow Riverwalk) is the first completed section of a 30-mile network of rail-trails being developed between the four communities of Amesbury, Salisbury, Newbury, and Newburyport. The riverwalk will eventually connect with the Salisbury Point Ghost Train Trail.

The trail starts on Water Street in the Lower Mills district of downtown Amesbury. Approaching the trailhead, you'll first see the large Boston & Maine Railroad Depot and then the much smaller Salisbury Point Station, which was built in the 1870s by the rival Eastern Railroad. In the late 1800s and early 1900s, the local economy revolved around the carriage building, involving more than 100 businesses, including 26 manufacturing companies.

On display outside Salisbury Point Station are historical photographs of the mill yards, the railroad, and the 1915 Annual Town Bike Race, showing men riding through Amesbury on high-wheeled bicycles. The trailhead also marks the future site of the Amesbury visitor center and a carriage museum.

Location
Essex County

Endpoints
Water Street to Carriagetown Marketplace in Amesbury

Mileage
1.3

Roughness Index
1

Surface
Asphalt

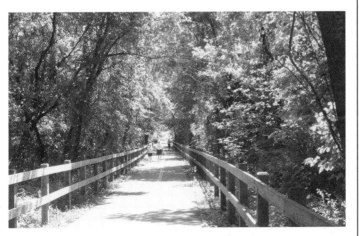

The Amesbury Riverwalk is part of an interconnected trail system being developed in the area.

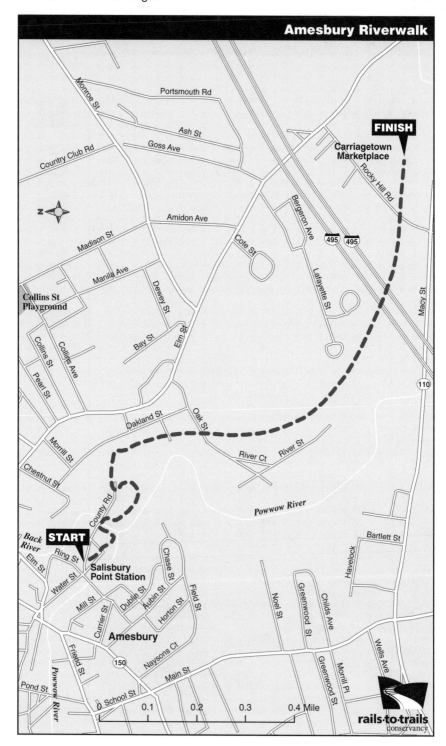

Amesbury Riverwalk

The first third of the riverwalk follows the bank of the scenic Powwow River. Keep watch for the area's abundant wildlife. The Powwow joins the Merrimack River in Amesbury, and both reach to the sea, making them rich habitat for a variety of birds and turtles, as well as beaver, mink, and fishers.

The trail briefly jogs across a road bridge via a sidewalk before it returns to the main railroad corridor and continues to parallel the river. Then the trail skirts a manufacturing company parking lot and loading dock before returning to a more typical, straight rail-trail route. The onward trail offers a peaceful walk through wooded areas and neighborhoods, with only two road crossings before reaching the trail's end at Carriagetown Marketplace.

DIRECTIONS

To reach the Amesbury trailhead, take Interstate 95 to Exit 58 for State Route 110 west. Turn right on Elm Street. In 2 miles, turn left on Water Street. The free municipal parking lot is on the left. The trail begins at the bottom of the hill.

To reach the Carriagetown Marketplace trailhead, take I-95 to Exit 58 for Route 110 west. At the second traffic light, turn right into the Carriagetown Marketplace parking lot. The trail starts on the far west end of the lot.

Contact: Alliance for Amesbury
5 Market Square
Amesbury, MA 01913
(978) 388-3178

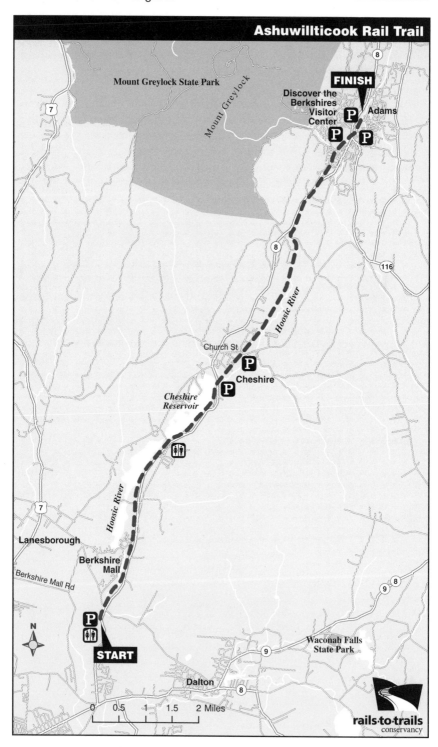

Ashuwillticook Rail Trail

Mount Greylock State Park

Mount Greylock

FINISH

Discover the
Berkshires
Visitor
Center

Adams

Hoosic River

Church St

Cheshire

Cheshire
Reservoir

Hoosic River

Lanesborough

Berkshire
Mall

Berkshire Mall Rd

N

START

Waconah Falls
State Park

Dalton

0   0.5   1   1.5   2 Miles

rails·to·trails
conservancy

Ashuwillticook Rail Trail

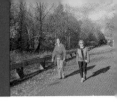

Nestled in the Hoosic River Valley between Mount Greylock and the Hoosac Mountains in Berkshire County, the Ashuwillticook Rail Trail takes its name from a Native American word meaning "the pleasant river between the hills." Gorgeous views of the mountains, lakes, and river, plus ample rest areas, make for a perfect day trip and contribute to this trail's popularity with locals and visitors to the scenic Berkshires.

Beginning at the Berkshire Mall in Lanesborough, the 11.2-mile route parallels State Route 8 through Cheshire on into Adams. Following the railroad corridor developed by the Pittsfield & North Adams Railroad in 1845, you'll pass lovely forested areas interspersed with lakes and small ponds.

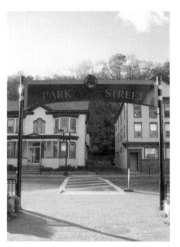

The Ashuwillticook Rail Trail at its connection to Park Street in Adams

At mile 2.7, the trail reaches some wetlands and the 418-acre Cheshire Reservoir, where you'll find no shortage of diversions. Pack a picnic, bring your binoculars for quality bird-watching, or cast a line from the side of the trail to reel in largemouth and rock bass, northern pike, and yellow perch.

As you approach Adams, the area's manufacturing history unfolds. You'll see mill buildings on the far shore of the Hoosic River, reflective of the area's manufacturing history. The trail parallels the town's delightfully restored main street, with interesting, quaint stores and eateries. Archways and banners throughout Adams sport a black bear riding a bicycle, a nod to both the trail and the resident black bear population.

Location
Berkshire County

Endpoints
Lanesborough
to Adams

Mileage
11.2

**Roughness
Index**
1

Surface
Asphalt

The trail's northern endpoint is in Adams at the Discover the Berkshires Visitor Center. If you're not up for the return trip by trail, you can catch a Berkshire Regional Transit Authority bus back to Berkshire Mall; each bus will transport two bikes. As an alternative, stop by the old railroad station building—now a charming pub—to refuel before starting back.

DIRECTIONS

To reach the Berkshire Mall trailhead, take the Massachusetts Turnpike/Interstate 90, to Exit 2 in Lee, then follow US Hwy. 20 west to US Hwy. 7 north for 11 miles to downtown Pittsfield. From the Park Square rotary, follow East Street/Merrill Road for 3.25 miles to the intersection of state routes 9 and 8. Continue straight through the intersection on Route 8 north for 1.5 miles to the Lanesborough-Pittsfield line. Turn left at the light for rail-trail parking at the Berkshire Mall.

To reach the northern trailhead from North Adams, take State Route 2 to Route 8 south for 5.5 miles to Adams. Follow the brown Ashuwillticook Rail Trail signs. Take a left on Hoosac Street, then an immediate right on Depot Street. Park at the Discover the Berkshires Visitor Center on the left. The trailhead is behind the visitor center.

Additional parking is available at Farnams Road and Church Street in Cheshire, and at Russell Field off Harmony Street in Adams.

Contact: Massachusetts Department
of Conservation & Recreation
251 Causeway Street, Suite 700
Boston, MA 02114
(617) 626-1250

Assabet River Rail Trail

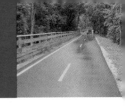

The Assabet River Rail Trail provides a forested escape from the surrounding urban bustle. Traveling 5.6 miles (with plans to expand it to 12 miles, the trail connects the towns of Hudson and Marlborough, and parallels the scenic Assabet River. The trail crosses the Assabet River five times, the last crossing on a refurbished, historical wrought iron railroad bridge. The 12-foot-wide corridor makes an excellent cycling route—just take care maneuvering between bollards located at the intersection of trails and roads; they are closer together than most.

The trail begins along Route 62 in Hudson, marked by a trailside, restored, 1921 blue caboose across the road from an ice-cream store. Look for the trailhead parking area.

Passing through downtown Hudson, the trail weaves through the awkward three-way intersection of Villa do Porto Boulevard, Broad Street, and the South Street extension. Returning to the rail corridor, you'll cross a wooden bridge, followed by more trailhead parking on

Location
Middlesex County

Endpoints
Hudson to
Marlborough

Mileage
5.6

**Roughness
Index**
1

Surface
Asphalt

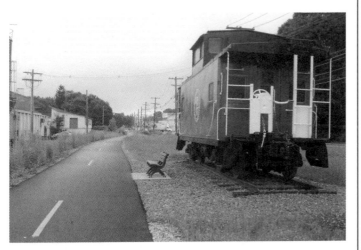

A restored railroad car reminds trail users of the Assabet River Rail Trail's history.

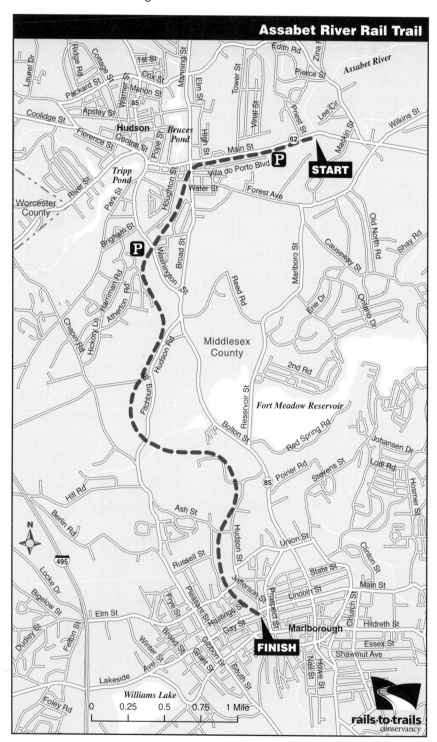

Assabet River Rail Trail

START

FINISH

Hudson

Marlborough

Middlesex County

Worcester County

Bruces Pond

Tripp Pond

Fort Meadow Reservoir

Williams Lake

Assabet River

N

rails·to·trails
conservancy

0   0.25   0.5   0.75   1 Mile

your right. The forested trail here provides a welcome buffer from the surrounding residential and urban landscape.

At mile 2.4, you'll cross the Marlborough town line through a tunnel. The onward trail skirts a main road north, passing the Boston Scientific medical research and corporate center before reaching Fitchburg Street. Be careful at this intersection, as there are no bike lanes and the traffic light cycle doesn't allow much time to cross.

Beyond the crossing, there are no bike lanes. Look for the trail sign after the intersection, and you will find yourself leaving the traffic behind. As the path diverges from the road, the adjacent, landscaped swathes on either side of the route shield trail users from the busy urban environment. Side trails connect to the Assabet along this stretch.

Eventually, the trail will extend to South Acton along the Marlborough Branch Railroad corridor, which connected the Fitchburg and Massachusetts Central railroad lines. The five communities along the corridor are working together to develop the rail-trail.

DIRECTIONS

To reach the Wilkins Street trailhead in Hudson, take Interstate 495 to State Route 62 toward Hudson. Once in town, continue through the rotary to the parking lot on Wilkins Street.

To reach trailhead parking in Marlborough, take I-495 to State Route 20/Granger Boulevard toward Marlborough. Turn left on State Route 85/Bolton Street, left on Union Street, then left again on Hudson Street. The parking lot is across from Kelleher Field and Jefferson Street.

Contact: Hudson Town Hall
78 Main Street
Hudson, MA 01749
(978) 562-9963

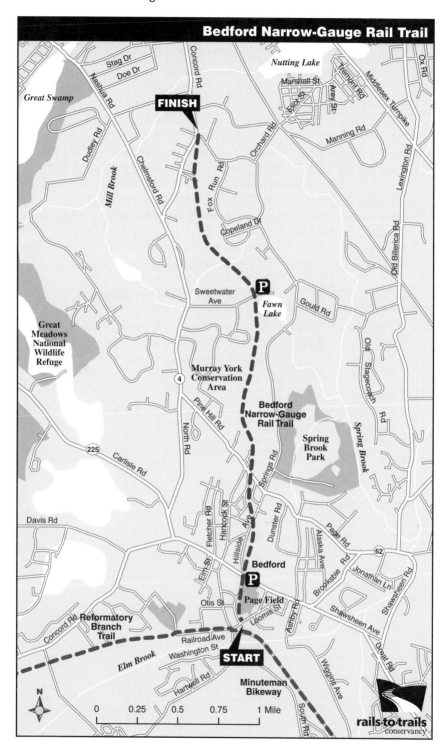

Bedford Narrow-Gauge Rail Trail

Bedford Narrow-Gauge Rail Trail

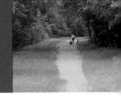

The Bedford Narrow-Gauge Rail Trail shares its trailhead at Depot Park in Bedford with the Minuteman Bikeway (see page 119) and Reformatory Branch Trail (see page 135). Serving mainly as a commuter route, this trail extends just over 3 miles north past woods and residences to the Billerica town line. It also makes a nice diversion for Minuteman Bikeway users looking to picnic at the York Conservation Area.

The trail follows the bed of the 1877 Billerica & Bedford Railroad, the nation's first 2-foot narrow gauge railway. In 1885, the Boston & Lowell Railroad built a standard gauge extension of the line. The Lexington Branch served five passenger stations—Bedford Springs, South Billerica, Turnpike, Billerica, and Bennett Hall. The railroad abandoned the extension in 1962, and the town of Bedford purchased it to create the trail. Cyclists should use either hybrid or mountain bikes, as portions of the route are surfaced with stone dust.

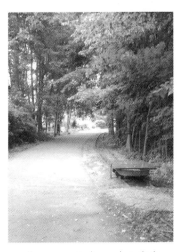

Narrow gauge tracks run alongside the trail.

Metal gates signal the start of the asphalt-paved trail at Loomis Street. Along the first mile to Great Pond, you'll pass the gardens at Memorial Park on the right, followed by a retail district. Use caution at the unmarked Great Road intersection. Beyond this crossing, the trail surface changes to stone dust.

A passenger station once stood at the intersection on Springs Road. Look for the electromagnetic "wigwag" (a railroad grade crossing signal) that once warned approaching motorists. Beyond the Pine Hill Road intersection, to the left of the trail, York Conservation Area

Location
Middlesex County

Endpoints
Bedford to Billerica town line

Mileage
3.1

Roughness Index
2

Surface
Asphalt, crushed stone, dirt

offers a welcome stop for a picnic on the green or a stroll around the pond. Bikes are not permitted, but you can explore the conservation area on foot.

Back on the Bedford Narrow-Gauge Rail Trail, and approaching its end, the trail becomes increasingly sandy. Metal gates at the Billerica town line signal where the trail ends abruptly. A private residential street follows the remainder of the railbed.

On weekends, consider returning to Bedford Depot Park for a tour of the charmingly restored freight house (open seasonally), which holds antique photos and railroad memorabilia.

DIRECTIONS

To reach the Bedford Depot Park trailhead from Boston, take Interstate 495 to State Route 3 south or I-95 to Route 3 north. From Route 3, take Exit 26 and follow State Route 62 west into Bedford. Trailhead parking is available.

Contact: Friends of Bedford Depot Park
120 South Road
Bedford, MA 01730
(781) 687-6180
www.bedforddepot.org

Cape Cod Rail Trail

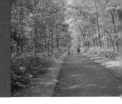

This 22-mile rail-trail serves up a genuine Cape Cod experience, stretching through quaint villages and along sandy beaches past a diverse landscape of salt marshes, pine forests, and cranberry bogs. The trail is paved, with few inclines, and trailheads sprinkled along the route offer restrooms, food, water, and swimming areas. You'll also find trailside shops where bicycle—and even handcycle—rentals are a breeze.

The trail follows the former Old Colony Railroad right-of-way from South Dennis to South Wellfleet, via Harwich, Brewster, Orleans, and Eastham. The railroad laid the tracks linking Boston and Sandwich in 1848, and by 1873, it had pushed all the way to Provincetown at the tip of Cape Cod. As the cape gained popularity with vacationers, more railroad connections were made to New York, Connecticut, and other parts of Massachusetts. Passenger service ceased in 1937; transport freight hung on until the mid-1960s. By 1978, the trail was in place, and vacationers once again hit the corridor—this time on foot, inline skates, and bicycles.

Near its western trailhead in South Dennis, the trail is at its busiest. The first 4 miles offer ample opportunities to picnic, indulge in ice cream, or detour to other trails and towns. From a large, unique bicycle rotary in Harwich, the

Location
Barnstable County

Endpoints
South Dennis to
South Wellfleet

Mileage
22

Roughness Index
1

Surface
Asphalt

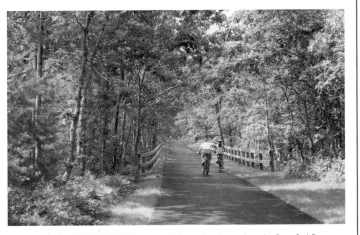

Popular Cape Cod Rail Trail follows a cool, forested pathway along the Cape Cod Bay.

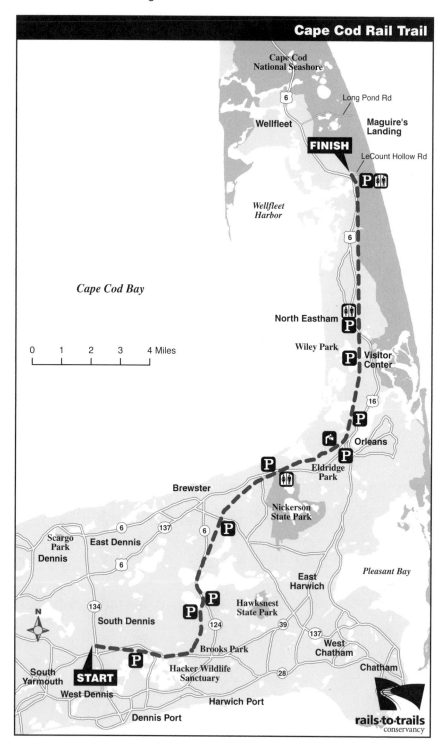

Old Colony Rail Trail continues through Harwich and the Hacker Wildlife Sanctuary and ends in Chatham. The beautifully landscaped rotary doubles as a gateway to the rest of the Cape Cod Rail Trail, providing a picnic area and trail information kiosks.

Heading north from the rotary, you'll soon be sailing along busy US Route 6 past glacial ponds. Along the way, you can pop into a quaint general store for a refreshment or take a break at a trailside picnic table.

At the trail midpoint near mile 11, you'll reach Nickerson State Park, which offers swimming pools, picnic areas, walking and biking trails, and restrooms. The forested trail here makes for a shady, cool ride.

Past Nickerson, the trail breaks and continues along the road for about a half mile and crosses a bridge before rejoining the corridor into the delightful town of Orleans. Boasting a range of restaurants and specialty stores, Orleans is a good place to stop for lunch. Also watch for the trailside water fountain and bike rental shop.

As you approach mile 16 along the Cape Cod National Seashore, be on the lookout for the Salt Pond Visitor Center, which houses a bicycle repair shop. The remaining miles of the corridor are lightly forested in trees and shrubs that have adapted to drier, sandier conditions. This stretch offers public camping facilities and coastal overlooks.

At trail's end, the Wellfleet trailhead provides a parking area and basic restroom. The town itself occupies a narrow strip of the cape, flanked by the Atlantic Ocean and Cape Cod Bay. It's well worth continuing another mile on Long Pond Road to Maguire's Landing, where you can look for shells on the lovely beach, take a dip in the Atlantic, or simply enjoy the rewarding ocean view.

DIRECTIONS

The Cape Cod Rail Trail is in the mid-cape area in southeastern Massachusetts. Free parking is available at several locations, including the trailhead on Route 134 in South Dennis and the trailhead on LeCount Hollow Road in South Wellfleet.

To reach the South Dennis trailhead, take US Hwy. 6 to Exit 9 and head south on State Route 134 past Patriots Square Plaza and Cumberland Farms. The trailhead parking area is on the left, about a half mile south of the exit.

Contact: Nickerson State Park
Massachusetts Department
of Conservation & Recreation
251 Causeway Street, Suite 600
Boston, MA 02114
(617) 626-1250

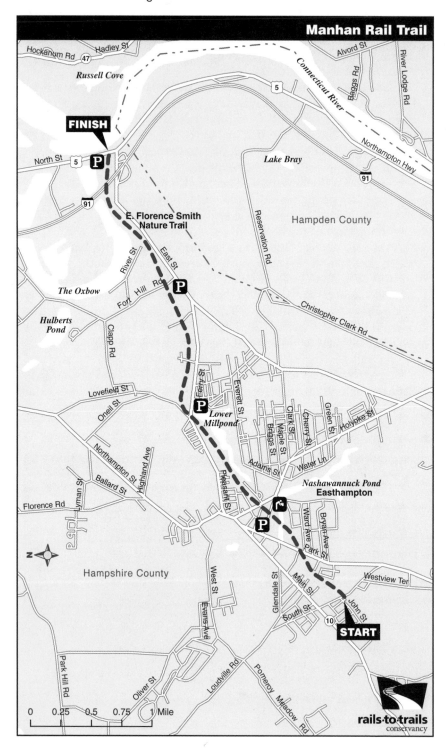

Manhan Rail Trail

The Manhan Rail Trail wends its way through Easthampton, a typical New England factory town brimming with commerce and community, as well as historical and natural sites galore. Located in the Pioneer Valley of western Massachusetts, the 4-mile trail follows two former railroad corridors: New Haven Railroad's Canal Division, and Boston & Maine Railroad's Mount Tom Branch. These lines used to compete for business from the thriving textile mills, but by the 1970s, changes in environmental laws and relocation of the industry to southern states led to a decline in manufacturing and subsequently the rail.

Starting from South Street, the trail is characterized by a forested landscape, which makes for a cool, shady ride. About a half mile from the trailhead, an underpass provides student commuters access to the private Northampton Williston School. This part of the Manhan trail passes behind residential areas; entrances to the trail from neighborhood streets will give you a sense of the rail-trail's popularity. At 0.9 mile, you'll find trailhead parking and a water fountain on your right, followed soon after by the colorful *Manhan Rail Trail Millennium*

Location
Hampshire County

Endpoints
South Street
to North Street,
Easthampton

Mileage
4.2

**Roughness
Index**
1

Surface
Asphalt

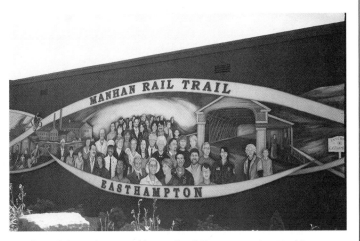

This trailside mural was painted by artist Nora Valdez to capture the spirit of the Easthampton community.

Mural. The colorful example of public art stands opposite an old train depot.

Crossing Ferry Street in Easthampton's business district, the trail veers due east on the old Boston & Maine corridor, soon opening up to a spectacular view of a Connecticut River tributary. Old mill buildings flank the trail to the left. On the right, a skateboard and basketball park with picnic tables is under construction. Just past the park, you'll find additional trail parking and access.

The trail passes more old mill buildings before reaching a scenic overlook of an oxbow in the Connecticut. This stretch keeps birders busy. Off to the right is the E. Florence Smith Nature Trail. Managed by the Pascommuck Conservation Trust, this short spur leads to the site of a 1704 conflict between settlers and Native Americans.

Nearing trail's end, you'll pass a residential area with parking and trail access on the right, and lovely open meadows on either side. You'll soon emerge at the small trailhead parking area on North Street/US 5.

The trail will eventually connect with the Norwottuck Rail Trail (see page 129) and Northampton Bikeway (see page 125).

DIRECTIONS

To reach trailhead parking on Ferry Street from the Massachusetts Turnpike/Interstate 91, take I-91 north to Exit 18 and head south on US Hwy. 5 to Easthampton. Turn right on East Street, then right again on Ferry Street. The trail crosses Ferry Street near the Pleasant Street intersection. Look for the parking lot on your left.

Contact: City of Easthampton
50 Payson Avenue
Easthampton, MA 01027
(413) 529-1460
www.manhanrailtrail.org

Marblehead Rail Trail

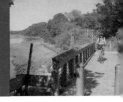

Shaped like a Y, this 4.1-mile rail-trail connects two seaside towns. From the trail junction in quaint Marblehead, one branch meanders through conservation areas and past harbor overlooks to Salem, notorious for its 1692 witch trials. The second branch offers a longer route heading toward Swampscott through Marblehead's residential areas, offering a more local look at this seaside community.

The intersection of Bessom Street and Roundhouse Road in central Marblehead marks the apex of the trail, and a good starting point. Follow the

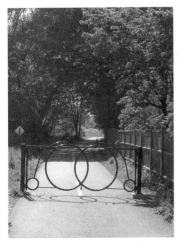

Artistic gates bar motorized traffic on the Marblehead Rail Trail.

sandy path on the west side of Bessom Street a quarter mile to the trail junction beside a fenced utility yard. Time to choose: to the right lies Salem, while the left branch leads down the coast toward Swampscott.

The branch toward Salem begins with a natural, sandy surface, and soon enters Hawthorn Pond Conservation Area, a 9.8-acre preserve with marshes, ponds, streams, and four interconnected nature trails. Take care as you emerge from the conservation area on West Shore Drive, as traffic can be heavy.

Up next is Wyman Woods Conservation area, a 33.5-acre mix of wetlands and mature forests that gives way to beautiful views of Salem Harbor. On warm days, trail users can hike down a sandy path to the water's edge for a refreshing dip or stop along the wooden railroad bridge for a particularly inspiring view of the harbor.

Entering Salem, the trail crosses Route 114; use caution at this major artery. Beyond, artistic gates modeled after antique high-wheel bicycles mark the path, and the

Location
Essex County

Endpoints
Marblehead to Salem and Swampscott

Mileage
4.1

Roughness Index
2.5

Surface
Asphalt, gravel, sand

115

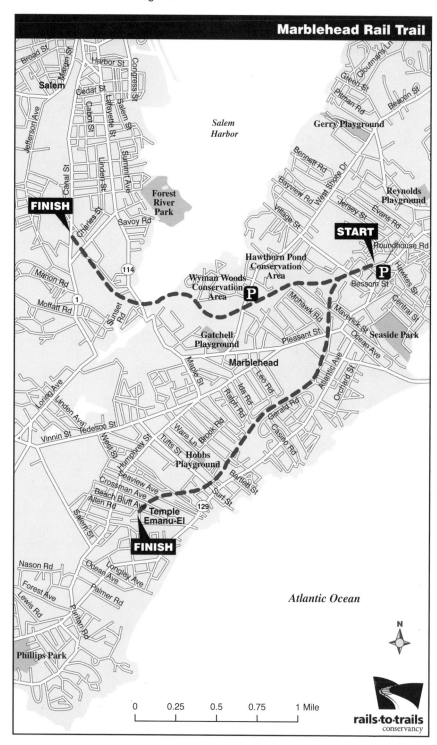

Marblehead Rail Trail

Salem

Salem
Harbor

Gerry Playground

Reynolds
Playground

FINISH

Forest
River
Park

START

Roundhouse Rd

Hawthorn Pond
Conservation
Area

Wyman Woods
Conservation
Area

Gatchell
Playground

Seaside Park

Marblehead

Hobbs
Playground

Temple
Emanu-El

FINISH

Phillips Park

Atlantic Ocean

N

0   0.25   0.5   0.75   1 Mile

rails·to·trails
conservancy

surface switches to smooth asphalt. You'll soon pass Salem State College, then enter a commercial area. The trail ends at Canal Street.

The alternative branch of the trail toward Swampscott also begins on a natural sand and gravel surface. Crossing Pleasant Street, you'll pass the public high school, where ball fields and playgrounds offer ample open space for a quick stretch or a relaxing break. Students use the route as a commuter corridor.

From the high school, the asphalt trail continues along a raised corridor through residential areas, with plenty of paved access roads to Marblehead beaches. The trail ends at the Temple Emanu-El parking lot.

DIRECTIONS

To reach the main trailhead, take State Route 128 to Exit 25 and head south on State Route 114 south to Marblehead. In town, 114 becomes Lafayette Street and then Pleasant Street. Follow Pleasant Street into town, then turn left on Bessom Street. Just past the shopping center on the right, take your first right turn onto Roundhouse Road. The trailhead is across the street.

Contact: Marblehead Department of Recreation
10 Humphrey Street
Marblehead, MA 01945-1906
(781) 631-3350

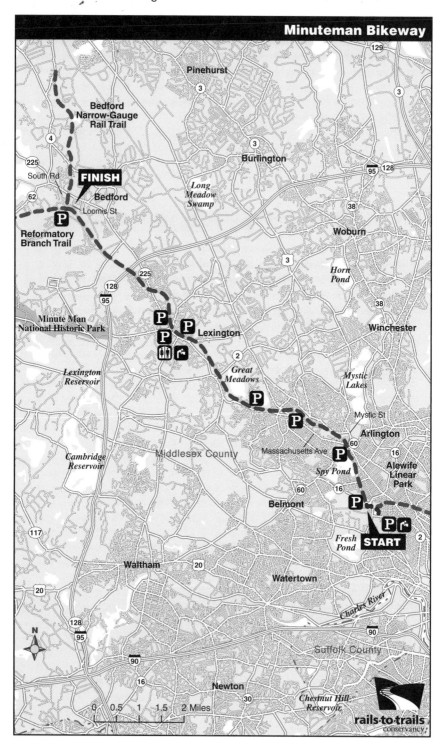

Minuteman Bikeway

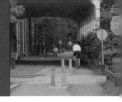

Y ou won't get lonely on the Minuteman Bikeway. The 11-mile rail-trail through suburban Boston is one of New England's most popular trails. Warm summer weekends in particular bring folks of all ages and abilities elbow to elbow along the asphalt bikeway.

The corridor boasts more than a vibrant present. It has a storied past that includes, as the name implies, a role in Revolutionary War times. The trail travels through the area where the Revolutionary War began in April 1775. In 1846, the Lexington & West Cambridge Railroad built and started service on the line. The blizzard of 1977 halted passenger service for good, and the demise of freight service followed in 1981. In 1991, the line was "railbanked" by federal law, making it possible to transform the line into a rail-trail while preserving future railroad opportunities. Just a year later, Rails-to-Trails Conservancy and the communities along the route celebrated the opening of the Minuteman Bikeway as the country's 500th rail-trail. By 1998, the Minuteman Bikeway was extended from downtown Arlington to the Alewife T-station in Cambridge. In 2000, the White House recognized the trail as a Millennium Trail (a program of

Location
Middlesex County

Endpoints
Alewife T-station
in Cambridge to
Bedford

Mileage
10.4

**Roughness
Index**
1

Surface
Asphalt

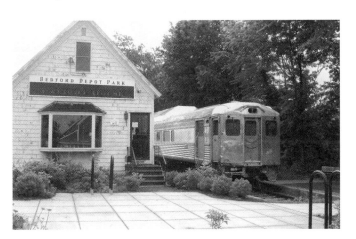

The Bedford Depot Park marks the trail's northern trailhead, where you can continue onto the Reformatory Branch Trail.

the Clinton Administration that noted outstanding trails in honor of the millennium), solidifying its reputation as a premier recreation and transportation route.

Although most users know the entire route as simply the Minuteman Bikeway, there are actually several connecting trails that can lead you from Somerville to downtown Concord.

Coming from Boston, you have the option to hop the Red Line subway to Alewife T-station, where the Minuteman begins. To add 1.5 miles to your route, jump off at Davis Square Station and take the Alewife Linear Park (see page 95) to the Minuteman.

On the Minuteman Bikeway traveling north into Arlington, you'll begin to understand why this trail is popular with pleasure-seekers and commuters alike. Heading northeast from Cambridge, the bikeway connects Arlington, Lexington, and Bedford, easing access to neighborhoods, schools, and such natural areas as Spy Pond and Great Meadows. Its paved, flat surface is a bicycle commuter's dream come true.

At mile 1.5, the trail seems to dead-end at Swan Place in Arlington. Here, you'll take a very short on-road jog; sidewalks are available for those uneasy with road cycling. Turn right on Swan Place, proceed to Massachusetts Avenue, then turn left and look for the Cyrus E. Dallin Art Museum on your right. A set of old train tracks crosses in front of the museum. Follow these tracks with your eyes, and you'll spot the onward bikeway, across Mystic Street.

Back on the trail, you'll soon reach the Lexington Visitor Center, which provides information about local attractions and historical sites.

Farther north, the wooded corridor grows more peaceful before reaching the trail's end at Bedford Depot Park. You can end your journey here or push on to the Reformatory Branch Trail (see page 135) by following Loomis Street to where it curves and the 4.5-mile trail picks up. The Reformatory Branch Trail will lead you on a natural surface path through several protected wetlands to its western trailhead in Concord.

DIRECTIONS

To reach the Cambridge trailhead by subway, take the Red Line to the Alewife T-station. Bicycles are permitted on subways during off-peak hours on weekdays or all day on weekends.

To reach the Cambridge trailhead by car, take Interstate 95 to Exit 29A and head east on the Concord Turnpike/State Route 2 toward Arlington and Cambridge. At the end of the turnpike, bear right on Alewife Brook Parkway, then turn right on Cambridge Park Drive to the station. The trailhead is west of the station; park in the adjacent garage. For more information visit www.mbta.com.

To reach the Bedford trailhead, take I-95 to Exit 31B and head north toward Bedford on State Route 4/225. Drive 1.1 miles, then turn left on Loomis Street. The trailhead is at the South Road intersection, beside Bedford Depot Park.

Contact: Arlington Bicycle Advisory Committee
Town Hall Annex
730 Massachusetts Avenue
Arlington, MA 02476
(781) 316-3090
www.minutemanbikeway.org

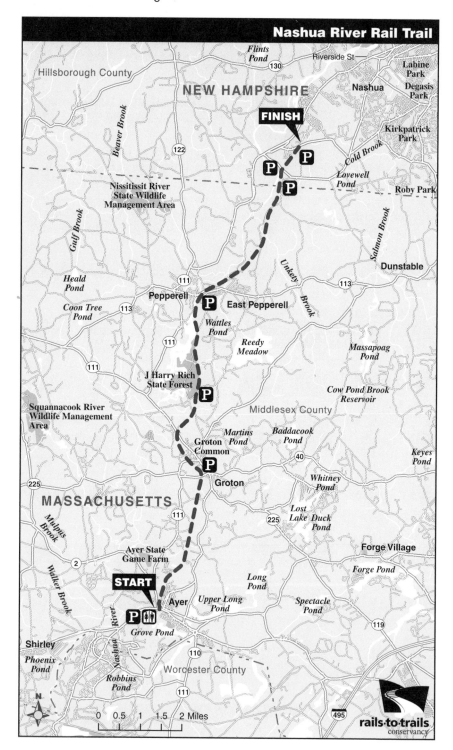

Nashua River Rail Trail

Nashua River Rail Trail

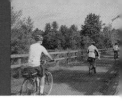

The Nashua River Rail Trail is a beautiful, peaceful, rural trail extending through the Massachusetts communities of Ayer, Groton, Pepperell, and Dunstable on into Nashua, New Hampshire. In autumn it provides a spectacular platform for viewing the colorful changing leaves. Over the 7 miles between Groton Center and Dunstable, a 5-foot-wide gravel equestrian path parallels the trail.

The 12.3-mile trail begins in downtown Ayer, across from the commuter rail station, where parking and restrooms are available. Leading north through residential Ayer, the route soon follows a rural, tree-lined corridor. Two miles into your journey, you'll reach Groton School Pond. Pause here at charming granite seating areas to watch for wildlife, particularly the industrious beavers that have built their lodge on the pond.

At the trail midpoint, you'll reach a small parking lot at Nod Road. Beyond, the trail skirts J. Harry Rich State Forest and the Nashua River, the latter visible to the west en route to New Hampshire.

A small retail and restaurant district hails your arrival in Pepperell. On a hot summer day, stop for an ice

Location
Middlesex County

Endpoints
Ayer to Nashua,
New Hampshire

Mileage
12.3

**Roughness
Index**
1

Surface
Asphalt

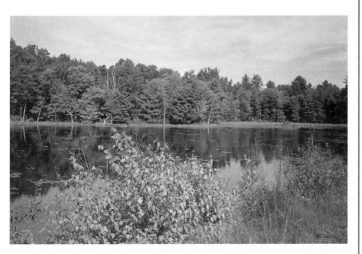

The Nashau River Rail Trail is one of several New England trails that cross state borders.

123

cream before continuing north to Dunstable, where you'll cross the border into New Hampshire.

The trail continues a short way into Nashua, ending at a large trailhead parking lot. Residential development on the corridor has severed the connection between the Nashua River Rail Trail and the 1.3-mile Nashua Heritage Rail Trail, which stretches east to Nashua City Hall. To reach the western trailhead from the parking lot, go straight on Countryside Drive and turn right on State Route 111/West Hollis Street. Turn left at the light on Riverside Street and follow it to the Nashua High School South playing fields. A trail here leads through Mine Falls Park to the park exit at Whipple Road. Follow Whipple to Simon Street, turn right, and continue to Will Street, where you'll turn left. The trailhead lies halfway down this street on the right.

DIRECTIONS

To reach the Ayer trailhead, take Interstate 495 to Exit 29 and head west on State Route 2 to Exit 38B for State Route 111 north. From the rotary, continue on 111 north through Ayer Center and the downtown shopping district till you see the trail from the road (still 111 north). For trailhead parking, take the first right past the trail, followed by another right into the lot.

To reach the Nashua, New Hampshire, trailhead, take US Hwy. 3 north to Exit 5W toward State Route 111A west toward Pepperell, Massachusetts. Follow it to Route 111 west. Turn left onto Countryside Drive. Follow it to the end to reach the trailhead. Trail parking is across the street in the parking lot.

Contact: Willow Brook State Forest
599 Main Street
West Townsend, MA 01474
(978) 597-8802
www.mass.gov/dcr/parks/northeast/nash.htm

Northampton Bikeway

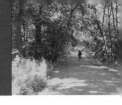

In central Massachusetts, the Northampton Bikeway runs 2.6 miles between Northampton and the Look Memorial Park in Florence. Whether you start your trip from either trailhead or from one of the many informal access points along the route, this well-maintained rail-trail is perfect for a fresh-air outing in a relaxed setting. It also serves as a vital commuter route, offering a convenient connection between the residential areas of Florence and downtown Northampton.

From the end of State Street in vibrant downtown Northampton, the trail leads west through residential and light commercial areas, passing several bed-and-breakfasts. If time permits, check out Main Street's architectural jewels, such as the Academy of Music and the county courthouse, as well as its many boutiques, restaurants, pubs, and coffee shops.

En route to Florence, forested stretches add to the trail's attractive, tranquil nature. You'll emerge at 150-acre Look Memorial Park, which provides ample paid parking. You'll also find picnic tables, a swimming pool, a playground, restrooms, tennis courts, and paddleboat

Location
Hampshire County

Endpoints
Northampton to Florence

Mileage
2.6

Roughness Index
1

Surface
Asphalt

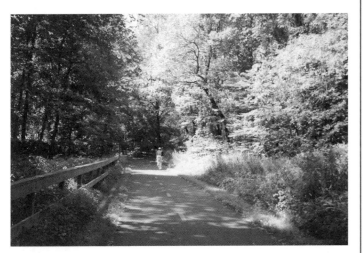

Despite passing through some neighborhoods and light commercial areas, the Northampton Bikeway makes for a tranquil trip.

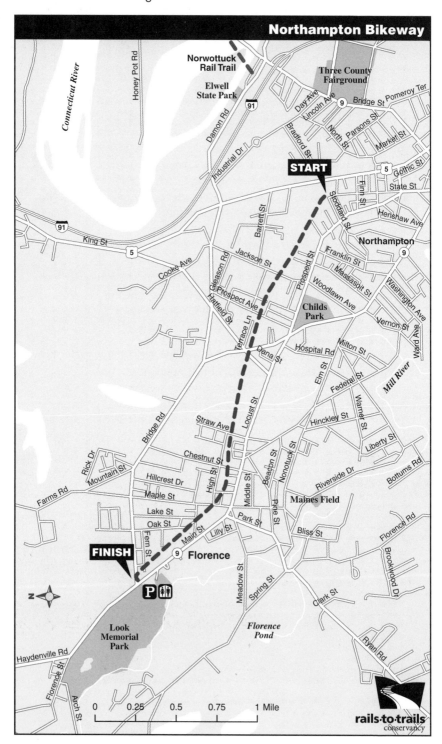

Northampton Bikeway

rentals. To use one of the picnic tables, you'll need to purchase a permit from the visitor center.

Crews are constructing a connecting spur to the 10-mile Norwottuck Rail Trail (see page 129), which stretches from Elwell State Park east through Hadley to Amherst.

DIRECTIONS

To reach the Northampton trailhead, take Interstate 91 to Exit 19 and head west on Damon Road. After about a block, turn left on US Hwy. 5/King Street. The trail intersects with King, just off the end of State Street.

To reach the Look Memorial Park trailhead from I-91 north, take Exit 19/Damon Road and follow signs to attractions. Cross State Route 9 on Damon Road and continue to the next light. Continue straight on Bridge Road for about 2 miles to the park. From I-91 south, take Exit 20, turn right at the light, and continue about 2 miles to the park.

Contact: Northampton Office of Planning & Development
210 Main Street
Northampton, MA 01060
(413) 587-1266
www.mass.gov/dcr/parks/central/nwrt.htm

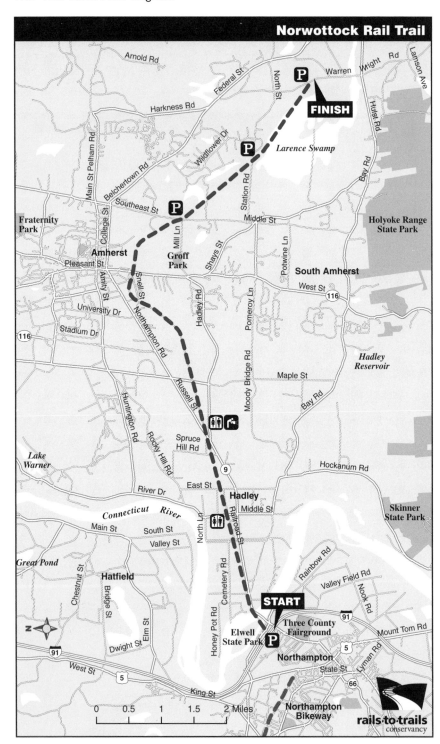

Norwottock Rail Trail

Norwottuck Rail Trail

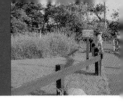

S tretching east from Elwell State Park, the 10-mile Norwottuck Rail Trail connects the towns of Northampton, Hadley, and Amherst. Part of the Connecticut River Greenway State Park, the route takes in a variety of landscapes, from rural farmland to residential neighborhoods and light industrial districts.

You'll set out across New England's longest river, the Connecticut, on a magnificent 1492-foot iron bridge. This span parallels Calvin Coolidge Bridge, named for the mayor of Northampton who would become the country's 30th president.

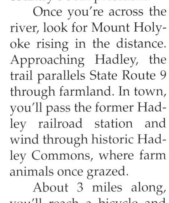

This trail travels through a sylvan setting and crosses a 1492-foot iron bridge over the Connecticut River.

Once you're across the river, look for Mount Holyoke rising in the distance. Approaching Hadley, the trail parallels State Route 9 through farmland. In town, you'll pass the former Hadley railroad station and wind through historic Hadley Commons, where farm animals once grazed.

About 3 miles along, you'll reach a bicycle and inline skate rental shop beside an ice-cream and smoothie bar. A half mile farther, just past the Route 9 underpass, is Pete's Drive-In, which offers a rest area and another chance for ice cream. Beyond it lies Hampshire Mall; shoppers will delight in direct bicycle access to the stores.

After the mall, the trail continues until the Belchertown trailhead, at which point you come to State Route 116. At 116, there is an opportunity to hop off the trail for a short trek north into Amherst, home to the University of Massachusetts and Amherst College. Just shy of downtown, a connector trail leads to the 2-mile UMass bikeway, a student commuter path.

Location
Hampshire County

Endpoints
Northampton to Amherst

Mileage
10

Roughness Index
1

Surface
Asphalt

The onward Norwottuck Rail Trail crosses beneath 116 to the Station Road trailhead and Amherst College on the left. Station Road used to mark the end of the trail, but today an extension stretches another mile east along an active rail corridor. Along the way, two trestle bridges carry you over Mill River and East Street, respectively, and you will find connecting trails to the Southeast Street access point and parking lot, as well as to hiking trails. The trail's final stretch skirts wetlands and ponds that promise excellent bird-watching. Along this section, the Caroline Arnold Walking Trail, which has a a bird-blind, can be accessed from the trail.

DIRECTIONS

To reach the Northampton trailhead at Elwell State Park, take Interstate 91 to Exit 19 and continue straight from the ramp onto Damon Road. After about a block, turn right into the trailhead parking lot at Elwell State Park.

Amherst offers a choice of parking locations. Parking is available near the town common and town hall, within easy reach of the Belchertown trailhead at State Route 116. To reach trailhead parking at Southeast Street and Mill Lane, follow State Route 9 to Southeast Street. Turn right and proceed about a mile. The Station Road trailhead lies a mile farther east; follow Southeast Street to Station Road and turn left into the parking lot.

Contact: Massachusetts Department of Conservation
& Recreation
136 Damon Road
Northampton, MA 01060
(413) 586-8706, Ext. 12
www.mass.gov/dcr/parks/central/nwrt.htm

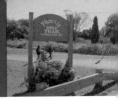

Opened in 1999, the Phoenix Rail Trail packs a surprising diversity in its 3.1 miles, passing through woodlands, salt marshes, farms, and commercial and residential areas. Tree-lined for much of its length, the path provides plenty of shade for a pleasant ride on hot, sunny days. Schoolchildren named the trail after nearby Fort Phoenix, within sight of which the first naval battle of the American Revolution was fought in 1775.

The trail begins in historical downtown Fairhaven, across from the old ferry terminal, where steamship passengers embarked for New Bedford before the bridge was built. The trail follows the path of the Fairhaven Branch Railroad, built in 1854, which stemmed off of the Cape Cod Branch Railroad. The Phoenix Rail Trail is the first section of a larger regional trail network that will eventually stretch from the Cape Cod Canal to Rhode Island.

The first half of the trail leads through Fairhaven's pleasant residential neighborhoods. Soon after setting out, you'll pass areas under redevelopment, including the site of the old Atlas Tack Company. The rail-trail's

Location
Bristol County

Endpoints
Fairhaven to Mattapoisett town line

Mileage
3.1

Roughness Index
1

Surface
Asphalt

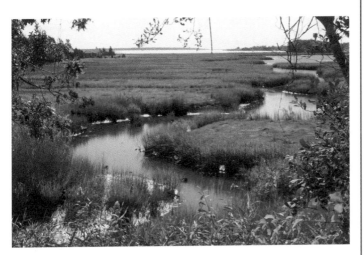

A view of a salt marsh from the Phoenix Rail Trail.

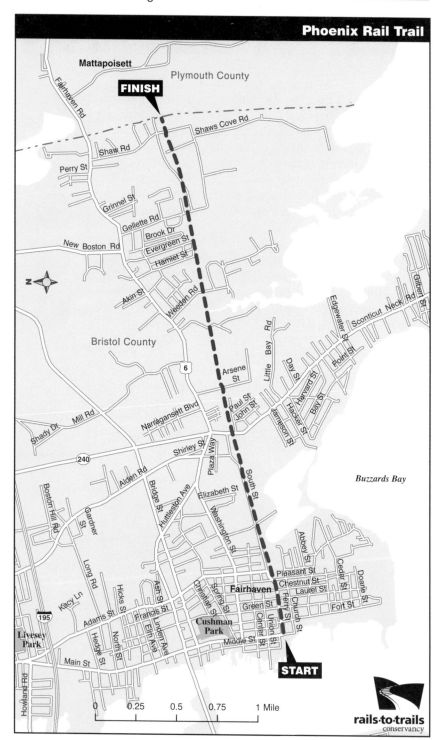

Phoenix Rail Trail

only major road crossing is the intersection with Route 240. From this point, the trail takes you through less populated areas, past farms with cornfields, and an outstanding vista of a salt marsh—a great place to spot birds and other wildlife. There, at approximately the halfway point on the trail, you'll note a short, marked spur trail called the Little Bay Loop Trail that takes off to the right. If you want to extend your ride, you can take the spur 1 mile to Buzzards Bay. At the junction of the spur trail, a kiosk displays a map of the trail and local area.

The trail currently ends at the Mattapoisett town line. While fairly short, the trail is quite popular among pedestrians and cyclists, and equestrians who utilize the grassy shoulder.

DIRECTIONS

To reach the Fairhaven trailhead, from Interstate195, take Exit 18 to follow State Route 240 south to US Hwy. 6 west. Follow signs to Fairhaven Center via Washington Street. Follow Washington Street east until you reach Main Street, turn left and continue a few blocks to the trailhead at the Ferry Street intersection.

Contact: Board of Public Works
5 Arsene Street
Fairhaven, MA 02719
(508) 979-4030
www.millicentlibrary.org/biketrail/bike1.htm

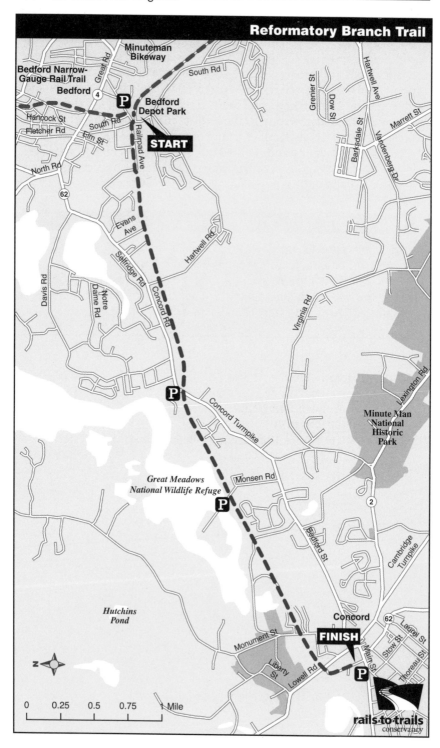

Reformatory Branch Trail

Minuteman
Bikeway

South Rd

Bedford Narrow-
Gauge Rail Trail
Bedford

Great Rd

Grenier St

Dow St

Hartwell Ave

Barksdale St

Vandenberg Dr

Marrett St

P Bedford
Depot Park

START

Hancock St
Fletcher Rd

South Rd

Elm St

North Rd

62

Evans
Ave

Hartwell Rd

Satfridge Rd

Davis Rd

Notre
Dame Rd

Concord Rd

Virginia Rd

Lexington Rd

P

Concord Turnpike

Minute Man
National
Historic
Park

Great Meadows
National Wildlife Refuge

Monsen Rd

P

2

Bedford St

Cambridge
Turnpike

Hutchins
Pond

Concord

62

Laurel St

Monument St

FINISH

Main St

Stow St

Thoreau St

Liberty
St

Lowell Rd

P

N

0   0.25   0.5   0.75   1 Mile

rails-to-trails
conservancy

Reformatory Branch Trail

The rugged and beautiful Reformatory Branch Trail meanders more than 4 miles through three natural areas: Elm Brook Conservation Area, Mary Putnam Webber Wildlife Preserve, and Great Meadows National Wildlife Refuge. It is the perfect route for escaping the city to rediscover nature.

Westbound from the Bedford Depot Park trailhead on Railroad Avenue, you'll first reach Elm Brook Conservation Area. Its 19.3 acres of protected wetlands and floodplain offer additional biking and hiking trails through an enchanting red maple forest.

Almost immediately after leaving the conservation area, you'll see signs for Mary Putnam Webber Wildlife Preserve. This 20-acre parcel is also mostly wetland and acts as a wildlife corridor for the many species that live within the surrounding wetland and woodland habitats.

At Concord Turnpike, the trail crosses a gravel parking lot and continues across the street behind the guardrail; it's a very narrow path here, but once you descend the small hill, it opens up again to a proper rail-trail. Regrettably, the wooden bridge that carried traffic over

Location
Middlesex County

Endpoints
Bedford to Concord

Mileage
4.5

Roughness Index
2

Surface
Dirt

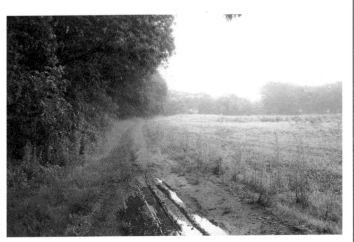

Linked to two other rail-trails, the Reformatory Branch Trail passes through several designated natural areas where wildlife sightings are common.

the railroad was removed in 1967. Be careful when crossing the busy turnpike, as drivers are not given warning of the trail crossing.

You will quickly arrive at Great Meadows National Wildlife Refuge. This massive freshwater wetland covers more than 3600 acres and stretches 12 miles along the Concord and Sudbury rivers. Birders take note: The National Fish and Wildlife Service, which manages the site, offers an annotated list of the area's 220 avian species. The refuge also shelters white-tailed deer, muskrats, red fox, raccoons, cottontail rabbits, weasels, amphibians, and several nonpoisonous snake species. Bicycles are not permitted on trails within the refuge; to explore, lock your bike to one of several trailside benches and take off on foot.

Back on the main trail, you'll leave natural tranquility behind as you draw closer to Concord. For approximately the last mile of trail, you will cross several roads; the trail ends shortly after crossing Lowell Road at the Concord River. The railroad corridor continues for another 2.5 miles, passing the reformatory for which it was named, but the bridge over the river is now gone.

DIRECTIONS

To reach the Bedford Depot Park trailhead, from Interstate 95/State Route 128, take Exit 31B for State Routes 4/225 north toward Bedford. After 1.1 miles on 225, turn left on Loomis Street. Loomis Street turns into Railroad Avenue; where the road bends to the right, look for the trailhead parking lot. You may park here or in the paved parking lot at the Minuteman Bikeway trailhead back on Loomis Street.

To access the trailhead in Concord, take Interstate 495 to State Route 2 east toward Concord. In town, turn left on State Route 2A east/Elm Street, which soon becomes Main Street. Park in the lot behind the Concord Visitor Center (64 Main Street), then follow the road directly behind the visitor center to the trailhead at Lowell Street.

Contact: Friends of the Bedford Depot Park
120 South Road
Bedford, MA 01730
(781) 687-6180

Shining Sea Bikeway

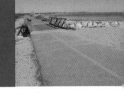

Curling more than 4 miles past woodlands, marshes, and salt ponds and seascape, the Shining Sea Bikeway is the only bikeway on Cape Cod to skirt the shore. Also called the Shining Sea Bike Path, the paved trail extends from Skating Lane in Falmouth to the Woods Hole Steamship Authority's site in Woods Hole, an historical seaside fishing village and home to an internationally known scientific community.

Rich in history, the bikeway follows prehistoric Wampanoag Indian trails. Members of the Algonquin nation, the peaceful Wampanoag were notable seafarers who thrived here on a plentiful diet of shellfish, fish, game, wildfowl, berries, roots, and nuts. In 1620, Wampanoag Chief Massasoit greeted Pilgrims, the first substantial wave of European immigrants. By the 1850s, Falmouth had become a destination for summer tourists, and the Penn Central Railroad soon stretched from Monument Village to Woods Hole, tracing the ancient Wampanoag trails.

The railroad stopped service in 1957, and within 20 years, the bikeway was built and dedicated as part of Falmouth's bicentennial celebrations. Today it serves as

Location
Barnstable County

Endpoints
Falmouth to Woods Hole

Mileage
4.5

Roughness Index
1

Surface
Asphalt

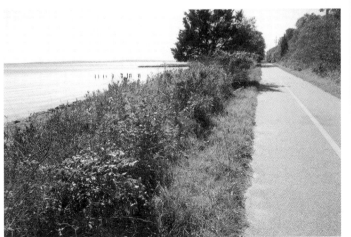

The Shining Sea Bikeway is aptly named—the views of Vineyard Sound are sparkling.

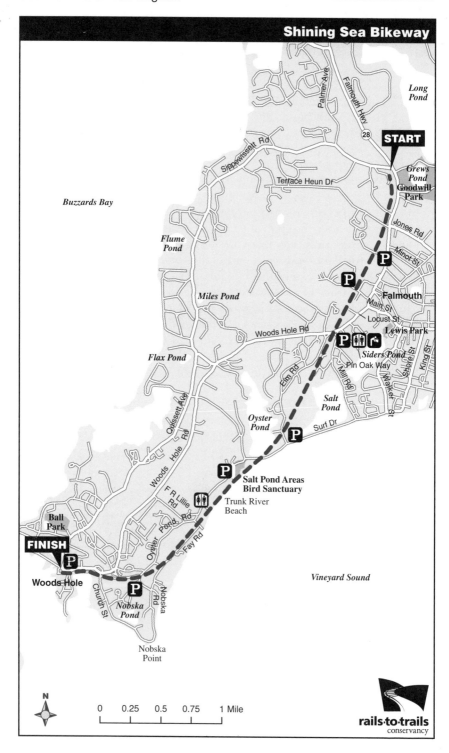

Shining Sea Bikeway

an inter-modal transportation link, connecting automobile, bus, ↳ and bicycle routes. Its name comes from "America the Beautiful," the famous poem by Katherine Lee Bates, a Falmouth native.

The route begins in Falmouth on Skating Lane in a residential and commercial district. As you follow the shaded path toward the water, you'll soon reach an information kiosk and spur path to the left for the Salt Pond Areas Bird Sanctuary. This 60-acre preserve between the bikeway and ocean offers a network of footpaths from which you can spot many species of shorebirds, as well as river otters and muskrats.

Soon after the sanctuary, the trail leaves the woods to reveal an expansive ocean view. This is truly the scenic highlight of the bikeway. Between the trail and the ocean lies Trunk River Beach, a barrier strand consisting of pebbles, cobbles, and sand. Pause here to breathe in the sea air or watch ospreys and herons glide over Vineyard Sound.

Continuing along the shore, the bikeway soon crosses the Woods Hole Steamship Authority parking lot. The trail ends in Woods Hole, affording you plenty of places to eat or shop.

DIRECTIONS

To reach the Falmouth trailhead from Boston, take Interstate 93 to State Route 24 south. Take Exit 14 for Interstate 495 south. Take I-495 to its end and continue on State Route 25. Follow signs for State Route 28 south to Buzzards Bay/Falmouth. Route 28 turns into a local road and leads you into Falmouth. Just before the ferry parking, turn right on Skating Lane. The trailhead is at the far end of the parking lot.

To reach the Woods Hole trailhead, follow the directions above, but continue to follow Route 28 past the ferry parking. Follow signs for Woods Hole (along Woods Hole Road), then follow signs to the Martha's Vineyard Ferry. Parking is available here, and the trail begins at the far end of the parking lot.

Contact: Falmouth Bikeway Committee
59 Town Hall Square
Falmouth, MA 02540
(508) 548-7611
www.town.falmouth.ma.us/depart.php?depkey=bike

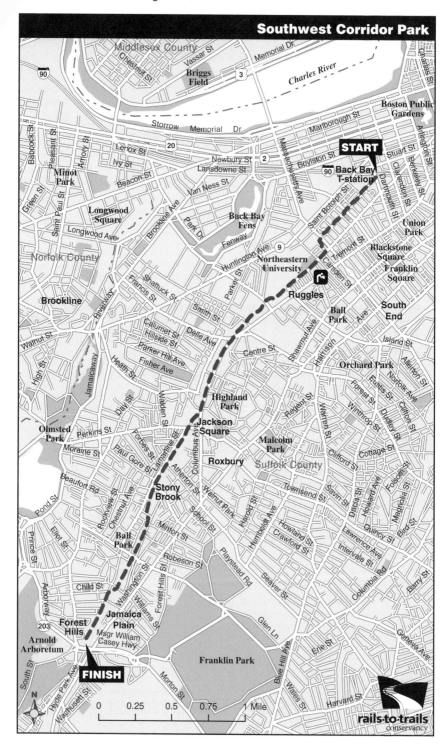

Southwest Corridor Park

Southwest Corridor Park

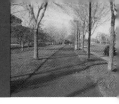

Southwest Corridor Park is a 3.9-mile linear park through the Boston neighborhoods of South End, Roxbury, and Jamaica Plain. A recreation and commuter route popular with walkers, runners, and cyclists, the corridor is a triumph of its surrounding communities, which rallied in the 1960s to prevent a 12-lane highway from flanking a subway line and instead created this 52-acre green space. The park parallels the Orange Line between the Back Bay and Forest Hills T-stations. Forest Hills connects to the Needham commuter rail line, while Back Bay is a stop on the Framingham/Worcester, Providence/Stoughton, and Needham commuter rail lines, as well as the Amtrak line.

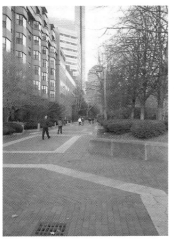

The Southwest Corridor Park is an important recreation and commuting route for local suburban neighborhoods.

The northern trailhead is across from the Back Bay T-station on Dartmouth Street, only blocks from Copley Square, the Boston Public Library, and commercial Newbury Street. Beginning between Neiman Marcus and Firefly Bistro, the trail winds its way between small residential South End side streets lined with historic brownstones. This skillfully designed section includes dog parks, playgrounds, neighborhood vegetable gardens, and basketball and tennis courts.

As the trail crosses West Newton Street, look up at the Prudential Center and John Hancock buildings, highlights of the Boston skyline. Where the trail crosses Massachusetts Avenue, glance right to spot Symphony Hall, home to the Boston Symphony Orchestra. As you approach Northeastern University's tennis courts, turn left and then right to remain on the path as it parallels

Location
Suffolk County

Endpoints
Back Bay T-station to Jamaica Plain, Boston

Mileage
3.9

Roughness Index
1

Surface
Asphalt

Columbus Avenue for a short stretch to Ruggles Station. Scattered along the corridor are more tennis courts, basketball courts, spray pools, street hockey rinks, and amphitheaters.

The path continues along Columbus Avenue, then cuts behind Jackson Square Station, where murals line the corridor to Center Street. If you're hungry, consider stopping in Jamaica Plain at City Feed & Supply, an excellent grocery and sandwich shop less than a block up Boylston Street from Stony Brook Station.

The trail ends just across Washington Street from Forest Hills Station, though you can extend your walk or ride into Arnold Arboretum, across South Street to the right of the station. The arboretum is part of landscape architect Frederick Law Olmstead's famous Emerald Necklace, a 1100-acre chain of parks that offers an alternate walking or bike route back downtown.

DIRECTIONS

Avoid driving in Boston by taking the T: Bicycles are permitted on subways during off-peak hours on weekdays or all day on weekends.

Back Bay T-station is on Dartmouth Street in Boston between Columbus Avenue and Stuart Street. There is no designated trail parking, but you'll find street and garage parking in the area.

Forest Hills station is just off the Arborway in Jamaica Plain, at the intersection of Washington Street, South Street, and Hyde Park Avenue.

Contact: Department of Conservation & Recreation
136 Damon Road
Northampton, MA 01060
(617) 727-0057
www.mass.gov/dcr/parks/metroboston/
southwestCorr.htm

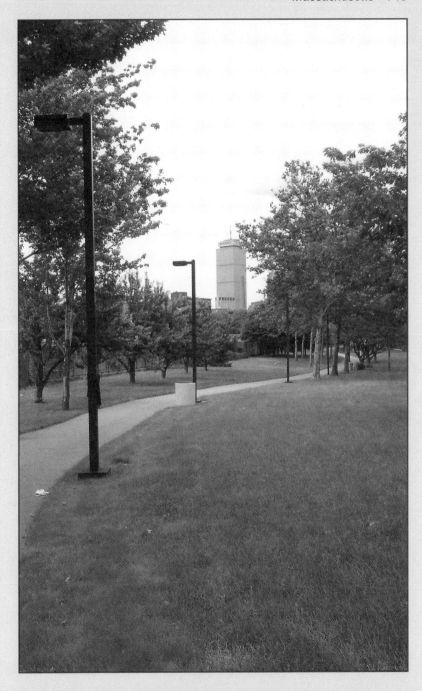

With connections to mass transit T-stations, the Southwest Corridor Park serves as an important link for Boston-area pedestrians and bicyclists.

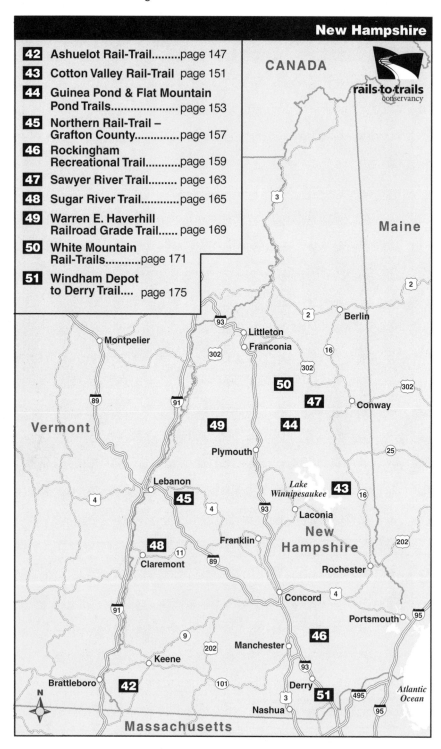

rails·to·trails
conservancy

CANADA

Maine

Vermont

Montpelier

Littleton
Franconia

50

47 Conway

44

Plymouth

49

Lebanon

45

Lake
Winnipesaukee **43**

Laconia

New
Hampshire

Franklin

48

Claremont

Rochester

Concord

Portsmouth

46

Manchester

Keene

Brattleboro **42**

Derry **51**

Nashua

Atlantic
Ocean

Massachusetts

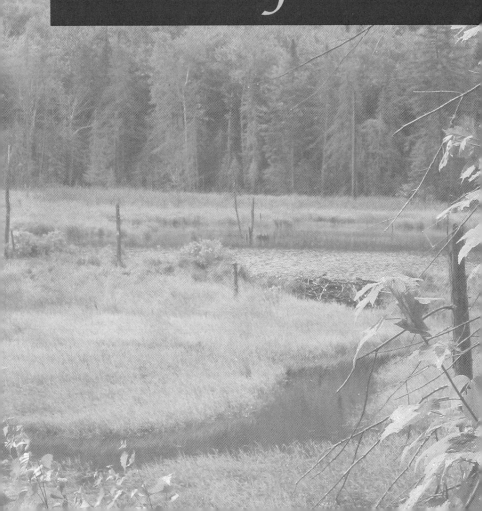

New Hampshire

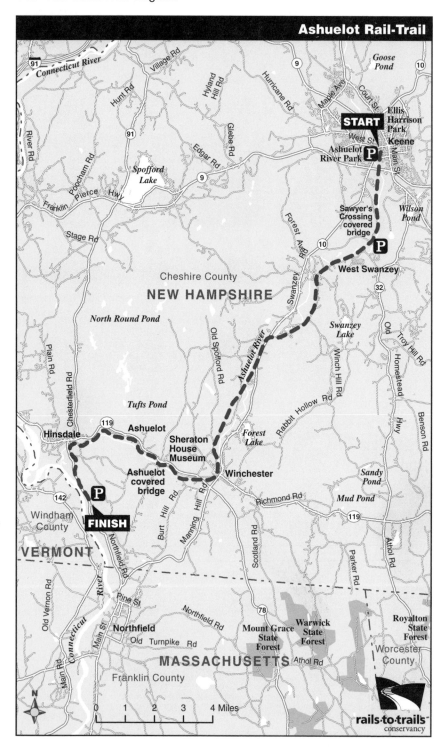

Ashuelot Rail-Trail

Ashuelot Rail-Trail

Given its covered bridges, historical aura, and abundant wildlife, the Ashuelot Rail-Trail (a.k.a. Ashuelot River Trail) has plenty lot to offer—as long you don't mind roughing it a bit. The trail surface of packed cinder, ballast, and dirt takes a pounding under heavy rains, which give rise to sandy, muddy, and even flooded trail sections.

The 21.2-mile route follows the corridor of the Ashuelot Railroad, which operated from 1851 to 1983, fostering the development of textile mills, wooden box factories, and leather tanneries in the region. Watch for the original granite mile markers, which pop up periodically along the trail.

From the trailhead on Emerald Street near Keene State College, you'll head south, tracing the Ashuelot River. Approaching West Swanzey, the trail passes near Sawyer's Crossing covered bridge, where you'll find a small parking area and a trail map. You'll soon reach a railroad trestle, marking your arrival in moose territory. Watch for moose tracks on the trail—similar to those of deer but twice the size—and if you do spot a moose, do

Location
Cheshire

Endpoints
Keene to Hinsdale

Mileage
21.2

Roughness Index
3

Surface
Cinder, ballast, dirt, sand

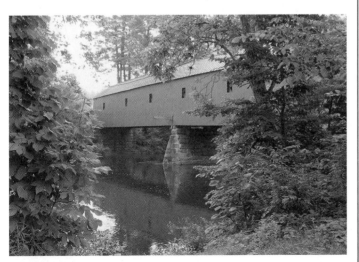

The Ashuelot Rail-Trail passes near Sawyer's Crossing covered bridge, one of two along the trail.

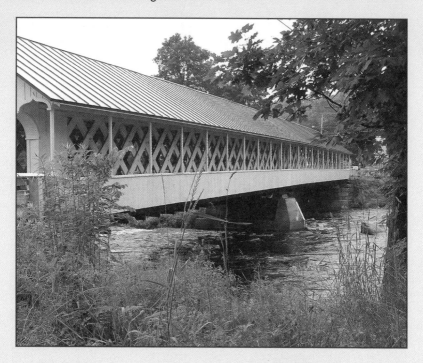

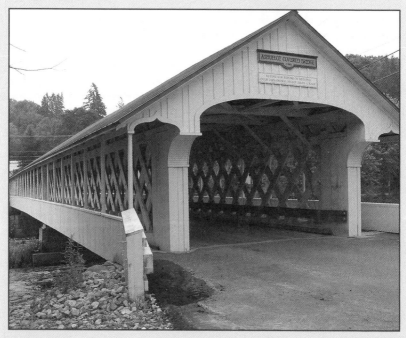

The Ashuelot covered bridge is considered one of New England's most sophisticated bridge designs.

not under any circumstances approach it, as they can be aggressive animals.

Next up is the historical town of Winchester, whose early settlers were repeatedly attacked and killed or taken captive by Indians. Following its burning in 1747, the town was rebuilt around its agricultural roots. Over the years, several small industries were established in Winchester. Graves & Company, one of America's first manufacturers of musical instruments, opened its doors here in the 1830s. The coming of the railroad brought still more industries and jobs to the region.

You can't miss Ashuelot's distinctive covered bridge, built in 1864 to bring wood across the Ashuelot River to fuel the burners of the railroad's steam engines. Considered one of New England's most sophisticated covered bridges, the span is 169 feet long, with intricate latticework and flanking sidewalks. A sign at each end of the bridge warns of a $5 fine for anyone riding or driving faster than a walk. Don't overlook the Sheraton House Museum on the other side of the trail.

The trail continues south, past old mills and rusting boxcars on sidings, to a high ridge with picturesque river views. Along the way you'll pass a railroad depot that's been restored and converted into a residence, complete with train cars on a siding. Near Hinsdale, the trail parallels State Route 63 past farmland. You'll emerge at a trailhead that links up with the Fort Hill Rail-Trail.

DIRECTIONS

To reach the Keene trailhead from Ashuelot River Park, turn left on West Street, right on School Street, then right again on Emerald Street. Parking is available in the shopping center lot directly across from the trailhead.

To reach the Hinsdale trailhead, follow State Route 63 for 2.1 miles south out of Hinsdale. The trailhead is on the right.

Contact: New Hampshire Bureau of Trails
PO Box 1856
Concord, NH 03302
(603) 271-3254
www.nhtrails.org

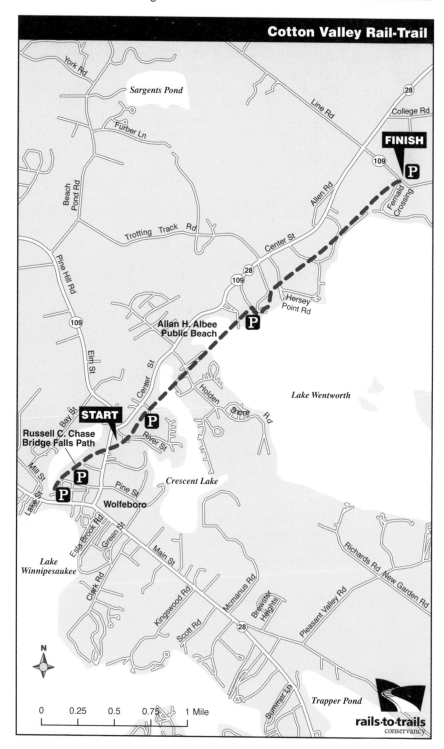

Cotton Valley Rail-Trail

Cotton Valley Rail-Trail

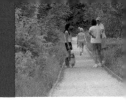

On the banks of Lake Winnipesaukee in central New Hampshire, Wolfeboro bills itself as "America's Oldest Summer Resort." Vacationers have been escaping to this quaint village since passenger rail service began in 1872. By the early 1900s, seven train stations dotted the 12-mile corridor east to Sanbornville.

Today, 3 miles of that route (with 3 more planned) serve as the multiuse Cotton Valley Rail-Trail (a.k.a. Wolfeboro–Sanbornville Rail-Trail). Volunteers from an association of railway motorcar owners work with a committee of local trail enthusiasts to plan and maintain the trail, with an eye to preserving the railroad's legacy. And in a unique rail-trail twist, sections of the trail actually run between the old rails, which are still in place and visible, though you cannot see the ties.

From the trailhead at the restored train depot on Railroad Avenue, the crushed stone Russell C. Chase Bridge Falls Path leads to the rail-trail proper. Be sure to pick up a copy of the trail brochure, which lists key points of interest marked along the way.

Causeways that lead across Crescent Lake, then along Lake Wentworth are another stunning feature on this trail—at times you're surrounded by water on either side,

Location
Carroll County

Endpoints
Railroad Avenue
to Fernald Station,
Wolfeboro

Mileage
3.2

**Roughness
Index**
2

Surface
Crushed stone,
sand

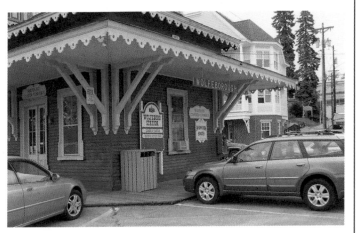

The quaint summer resort community of Wolfeboro was once serviced by the railroad on which the Cotton Valley Rail-Trail was built.

and the views are nothing short of spectacular. Wolfeboro's citizens use the trail for a variety of reasons: for commuting, for high school students to walk to school, and for recreation travel from the residential neighborhoods to the Allan H. Albee Public Beach on Lake Wentworth, where you, too, can pause to soak your feet or take a dip.

The onward trail skirts the lake for a little more than a mile to its current endpoint at Fernald Station. Leave time to take in Wolfeboro's wide range of shops and restaurants. Work is underway on the remaining few miles to Cotton Valley Depot.

DIRECTIONS

The Wolfeboro trailhead is at the restored train depot on Railroad Avenue, just west of the State Route 109 and State Route 28 intersection. Parking is available at the restored depot.

To reach the Fernald Station trailhead from Wolfeboro, head 3 miles north on State Route 28 north. Turn right on State Route 109. The trailhead is a quarter mile ahead on the right side of the road; park on the left.

Contact: Cotton Valley Rail-Trail Club
PO Box 417
Wolfeboro Falls, NH 03896
www.cottonvalley.org

Guinea Pond & Flat Mountain Pond Trails

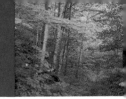

These connecting trails follow the bed of the old Beebe River Railroad up to Flat Mountain Pond, a large, remote pool high in the Sandwich Range Wilderness. This is a great trip for advanced mountain bikers; novice/intermediate bikers should expect a challenge. Hikers enjoy a relatively easy trek, as there's little gain in elevation.

Guinea Pond Trail begins at a metal Forest Service gate and climbs a dirt road 0.2 mile to the railroad bed. While the trail keeps to the railbed as best it can, at times you must detour around sections reclaimed by beaver ponds.

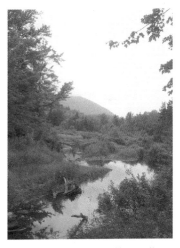

These two trails in White Mountain National Forest form a continuous path good for serious mountain bikers and casual hikers.

Just over a mile in, you'll pass a second metal Forest Service gate. Turn right at the Y-junction onto the well-trodden but unmarked path and ascend. After crossing three wooden bridges, the trail bends right to rejoin the railroad bed.

You'll soon reach the junction of the Mead and Black Mountain Pond trails. Continue straight on the Guinea Pond Trail. Following several wide stream crossings, you'll reach the marked 0.2-mile spur on the left to the pond itself.

The onward trail continues along the railbed to the 2.5-mile mark, where it detours again to avoid water (follow the yellow arrow to the left). This section is winding and rough, traversing large rocks and gnarly roots. The route finally rejoins the corridor after 0.2 mile and offers mostly smooth going to the Flat Mountain Pond Trail junction.

Location
Carroll County

Endpoints
Within White Mountain National Forest

Mileage
7.7

Roughness Index
3

Surface
Grass, dirt

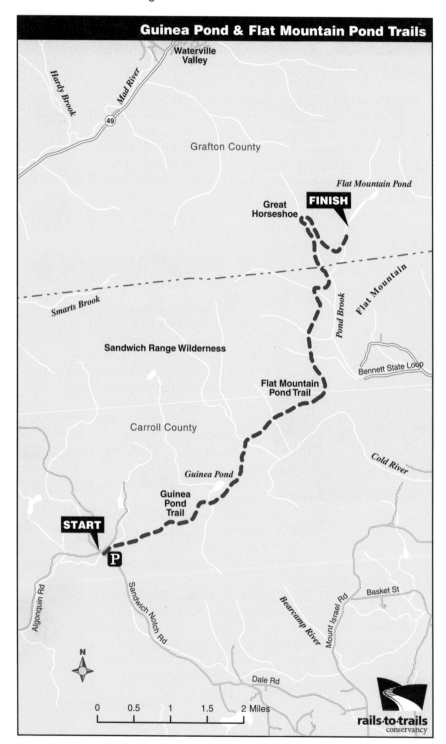

Guinea Pond & Flat Mountain Pond Trails

Waterville Valley

Hardy Brook

Mad River

49

Grafton County

Flat Mountain Pond

Great Horseshoe

FINISH

Smarts Brook

Pond Brook

Flat Mountain

Sandwich Range Wilderness

Bennett State Loop

Flat Mountain Pond Trail

Carroll County

Cold River

Guinea Pond

Guinea Pond Trail

START

P

Algonquin Rd

Sandwich Notch Rd

Bearcamp River

Mount Israel Rd

Basket St

N

Dale Rd

0   0.5   1   1.5   2 Miles

rails·to·trails
conservancy

The 4-mile Flat Mountain Pond Trail quickly gains elevation, soon passing the Gleason Trail junction. Watch for a sign on the left that marks the boundary of the Sandwich Range Wilderness; from here up to Flat Mountain Pond, the railbed doubles as that boundary. Note that bike riding is not permitted in the wilderness, so be sure to stay on the trail.

Drawing closer to the trail's end, you'll reach the Great Horseshoe, the sharpest turn on any of New Hampshire's old logging railroads. After navigating boulders, tricky streams, and other obstacles for about 2 miles, turn right at the trail junction and head toward the pond for beautiful views of Flat Mountain and Whiteface Intervale.

A shelter is available for those interested in overnight camping. Otherwise, retrace the Flat Mountain Pond and Guinea Pond trails to the trailhead.

DIRECTIONS

The trailhead is along Sandwich Notch Road, which is closed in winter. Only vehicles with good clearance should attempt this road. From Interstate 93, take Exit 28 to State Route 49 east toward Waterville Valley. After about 4 miles, turn right on Sandwich Notch Road and continue 5 miles until you see parking signs for the Guinea Pond Trail. Park down the dirt road on the right. From the parking area, walk or ride back to the road, turn right, and head downhill; the trailhead is on the left just over the bridge.

Contact: White Mountain National Forest
Pemigewassett Ranger District
1171 Route 175
Holderness, NH 03245
(603) 536-1315

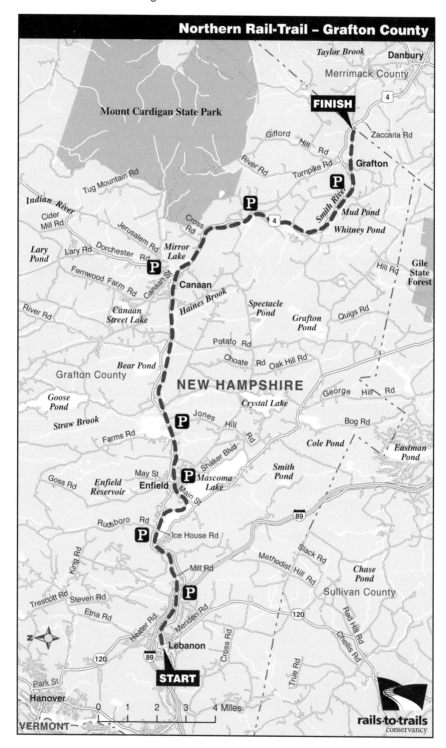

Northern Rail-Trail – Grafton County

Taylor Brook

Danbury

Merrimack County

4

FINISH

Zaccaria Rd

Gifford

Hill

Rd

River Rd

Turnpike Rd

Grafton

Mount Cardigan State Park

P

Smith River

Mud Pond

Tug Mountain Rd

Cross
Rd

4

Whitney Pond

Indian River

Cider
Mill Rd

Jerusalem Rd

Mirror
Lake

P

Canaan St

Haines Brook

Canaan

Spectacle
Pond

Grafton
Pond

Quigs Rd

Gile
State
Forest

Hill Rd

Lary
Pond

Lary Rd

Dorchester Rd

Fernwood Farm Rd

River Rd

Canaan
Street Lake

Potato Rd

Choate Rd Oak Hill Rd

Bear Pond

Grafton County

NEW HAMPSHIRE

George Hill Rd

Goose
Pond

Crystal Lake

Bog Rd

Straw Brook

Jones

Hill

Rd

P

Cole Pond

Eastman
Pond

Farms Rd

Shaker Blvd

Smith
Pond

Goss Rd

Enfield
Reservoir

May St

Enfield

P

Mascoma
Lake

Main St

89

Rudsboro Rd

King Rd

P

Ice House Rd

Stack Rd

Methodist Hill Rd

Chase
Pond

Trescott Rd

Steven Rd

Mill Rd

P

Sullivan County

Etna Rd

Meriden Rd

Cross Rd

120

Red Hill Rd

Chellis Rd

120

89

Lebanon

True Rd

N

Park St

Hanover

0   1   2   3   4 Miles

VERMONT

START

rails·to·trails
conservancy

Northern Rail-Trail – Graft County

Spanning the scenic Mascoma Valley of central New Hampshire, the Northern Rail-Trail stretches from Lebanon to the Concord town line. Local snowmobile clubs have decked the bridges and removed obstacles for winter use, and most of the 23.8-mile section between Lebanon and Grafton is now bikeable.

Plans are underway to build a four-season trail along the corridor in the Merrimack County towns of Danbury, Wilmot, Andover, Franklin, and Boscawen. Crews have already improved the 3.4 miles from Potter Place to Switch Road in East Andover, while improvements along an 8.3-mile section from Danbury to Potter Place are planned for 2010. Trail advocates will address Merrimack's remaining 23 trail miles as funds become available.

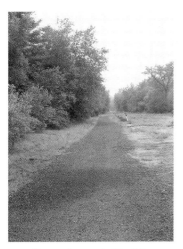

The meandering path of Smith River characterizes the majority of the Northern Rail-Trail – Grafton County.

From Lebanon, the trail follows the Mascoma River, crossing it seven times in just the first few miles. Benches are provided at several lovely overlooks. While this stretch is easily navigable in dry weather, heavy rains drench certain sections and put others wholly underwater.

Passing beneath Interstate 89, you'll enter a wooded river valley. Mill Road provides trail access, parking, and a small picnic area with tables. Beyond Ice House Road, the road parallels Mascoma Lake. Pause at one of the lakeshore benches to take in the views.

You'll soon encounter exposed rock along a dramatic cut—a reminder of the considerable effort expended to

Location
Grafton and Merrimack counties

Endpoints
Lebanon to Grafton

Mileage
23.8

Roughness Index
2

Surface
Crushed stone, cinder, grass, dirt, sand

construct this line. In 1847, native son Daniel Webster gave the keynote address in Lebanon at the railroad's grand opening.

Approaching Canaan, you'll cross a high bridge over the Indian River. Note the old depot, which has yet to be restored. Beyond town, the trail passes through two culverts. These are narrow with little headroom; cyclists should dismount and walk through.

Toward trail's end in Grafton, the general store beckons from across Route 4. This marks the last available parking on the improved section of the corridor, which ends at Zaccaria Road on the Merrimack County line.

DIRECTIONS

To reach the Lebanon trailhead near the Lebanon College campus, take Interstate 89 to Exit 18 and head south on State Route 120 toward Lebanon. The trailhead is at the intersection of Taylor and Spencer streets. If the trailhead parking lot is full, street parking is available.

To reach the Grafton trailhead, take State Route 4 east into town. Trail access lies opposite the general store. Park in the dirt pullout on the trail side of the highway.

Additional trailhead parking is available along Main Street off Route 4 in Enfield and at the end of Depot Street off Route 4 in Canaan.

Contact: New Hampshire Bureau of Trails
PO Box 1856
Concord, NH 03302
(603) 271-3254
www.nhtrails.org

Rockingham Recreational Trail

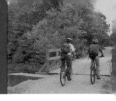

New Hampshire's largest city, Manchester, boasts relatively quick access to one of the state's longest rail-trails: the 26-mile Rockingham Recreational Trail (a.k.a. Portsmouth Branch). The rustic trail is rich in railroad structures, left over from a time when the extensive Boston & Maine Railroad network flourished with the growth of New England mill towns. The Rockingham Recreational Trail follows the Portsmouth Branch. Hurt by the mid-20th century decline in local manufacturing, the railroad faltered, and in 1988, the New Hampshire Department of Transportation purchased the Portsmouth Branch for conversion into a rail-trail.

The western trailhead lies just outside the Manchester city limits, right on the shore of Massabesic Lake, Manchester's public water supply. Much of the trail stretches through hardwood and conifer forests. In many places, standing water and bogs on either side of the railbed provide a breeding ground for mosquitoes. Bring insect repellent if you're on the trail between late spring and fall. If you're here when the snow flies, call out thanks to a passing snowmobiler: As with most trails

Location
Hillsborough and Rockingham counties

Endpoints
Manchester to Newfields

Mileage
26

Roughness Index
3

Surface
Dirt, sand

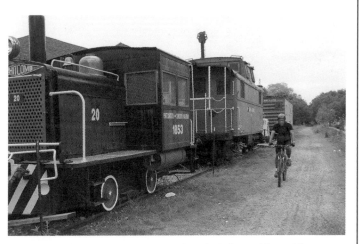

Near the trail's midpoint, railroad relics stand outside the Raymond Historical Society, which is housed in a restored train depot.

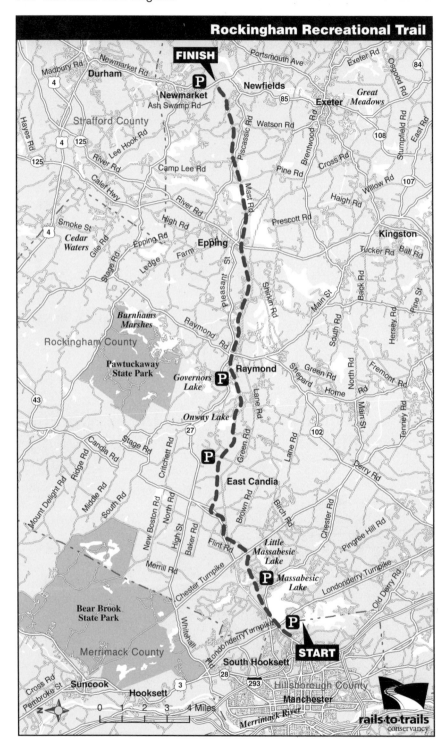

Rockingham Recreational Trail

in New Hampshire, the maintenance of this trail is taken on by local snowmobile clubs.

About 6 miles east of the trailhead, you'll encounter a narrow culvert beneath a road, with limited overhead clearance; consider dismounting and walking your bike.

In East Candia, a historical marker denotes the site of the demolished railroad depot. From this point, the trail again plunges into secluded woodland. The railbed rises above the forest floor at points, while other stretches thread through high-walled cuts blasted through New Hampshire's famous granite during the railroad's construction.

In Raymond, the local historical society has restored the train station. You can't miss the locomotive, caboose, boxcar, and work car on a siding between the trail and the station. Just beyond town, you'll cross an impressive railroad bridge and return to the wooded setting that typifies most of the route.

The Newfields railroad depot marks the trail's end.

DIRECTIONS

To reach the Massabesic Lake trailhead from Manchester, take State Route 101 north and east, then take State Route 28 south. After passing through a rotary, look for the Massabesic Lake boat launch on the left. The trailhead is at the boat launch.

To reach the trailhead in Newfields from the junction of state routes 108 and 85, head north on 108, cross the active rail line, and take the first left on Ash Swamp Road. Go to the end of the road and park at the old depot (do not park near the active rail line).

Contact: New Hampshire Bureau of Trails
PO Box 1856
Concord, NH 03302
(603) 271-3254
www.nhtrails.org

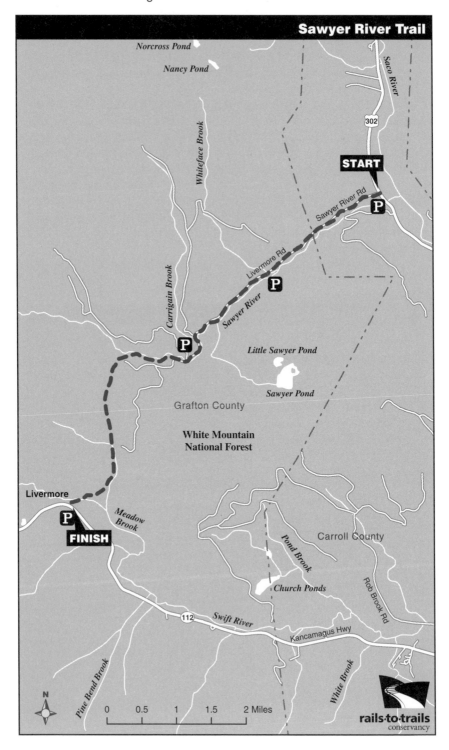

Sawyer River Trail

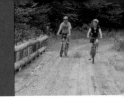

The Sawyer River Trail offers a memorable 7.5-mile journey through a pristine mountain valley. Following the old Sawyer River Railroad logging line, the trail is popular with mountain bikers and hikers for its combination of challenging single-track and dirt road sections.

There are a number of ways to attack the trail. The southern half of the 7.5-mile corridor, off the Kancamagus Hwy., is single-track. The northern half, near US Route 302, shares the corridor with Sawyer River Road, a quiet dirt road that closes in winter.

At its junction with US 302, Sawyer River Road ascends steadily at a manageable grade for 4 miles, following the Sawyer River. On your left at the start, watch for the abandoned sawmill village of Livermore, once-thriving hub of the Sawyer River Railroad.

The single-track section of the trail begins shortly after the metal Forest Service gate at the end of Sawyer River Road. If you're looking for a shorter, less-challenging trip, you can drive to this point of the trail and park in the parking area located nearby. Beyond the gate, turn

Location
Carroll County

Endpoints
Within White Mountain National Forest

Mileage
7.5

Roughness Index
3

Surface
Ballast, grass, dirt, sand

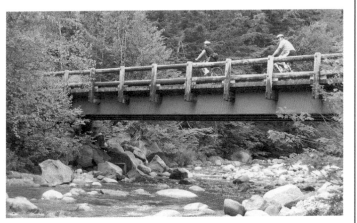

This trail has several river crossings, some of which have attractive spans like the one above—others you have to brave by boulder-hopping.

left at the fork and follow signs toward Meadow Brook. The trailhead will be on the right, around the bend.

The trail mostly sticks to the old railroad grade, detouring only to bypass sections flooded by beaver dams. While a generally flat grade affords hikers an easy walk through this stunning valley, the trail still provides cyclists some technical challenges. Watch for old train ties still in place, bridge supports for wooden railroad bridges, and other hints to the corridor's past.

Approaching the trail's end, you must cross the Swift River. There is no bridge, but boulders in the usually shallow river facilitate crossing. Use caution, particularly in the spring or after heavy rains, as high water can make the crossing difficult and dangerous. This is a great spot for lunch, however, and one of the best swimming holes around.

Beyond the river, you'll soon reach the Kancamagus Hwy. trailhead.

DIRECTIONS

To reach the northern trailhead, take Interstate 93 to Exit 35 and follow US Route 3 north to its junction with US Route 302. Take US 302 east through Crawford Notch. Sawyer River Road is on the right about 3 miles before the town of Bartlett. If you reach the Fourth Iron Tentsite, on your left, you've just missed the turn for Sawyer River Road. Park by the gate along US 302 or at pullouts farther up Sawyer River Road.

To reach the Kancamagus Hwy./Route 112 trailhead, take I-93 to Exit 32 to Lincoln and follow Route 112 east. Just beyond Kancamagus Pass, watch for a trailhead sign on the left. Park at the trailhead or along the road.

Contact: White Mountain National Forest
Pemigewassett Ranger District
1171 Route 175
Holderness, NH 03245
(603) 536-1315

Sugar River Trail

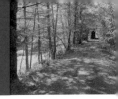

Also known as the Sugar River Recreational Trail, this picturesque 9.8-mile path stretches from Newport to Claremont along the banks of the Sugar River. Wildlife is abundant amid the secluded woodlands. Stay alert to spot deer, rabbit, beaver, raccoon, fox, wild turkey, or even an occasional moose around the next bend.

The trail's surface varies from firm cinder/ballast to soft sand. Traveling west from the Newport trailhead, the first 2 miles are particularly soft.

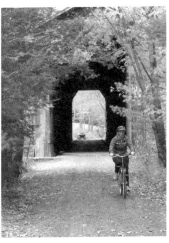

The Sugar River Trail boasts two historic covered bridges built by the Boston & Maine Railroad.

River crossings add to the Sugar River Trail's scenic allure, and covered bridge aficionados can anticipate a special bonus—two spans that once carried trains over the Sugar River: Pier Bridge (east of Chandler Station) and Wright's Bridge (named for S.K. Wright, who sold the right-of-way to the Sugar River Railroad). Both were built by the Boston & Maine Railroad and are on the National Register of Historic Places. Unlike covered bridges on New England roadways, these are much narrower and taller, with 21 feet of vertical clearance.

Additionally, the trail has nearly a dozen other bridges, ranging from small wooden plank structures to steel truss bridges that span the Sugar River and its side streams.

If the trail inspires you to see more of the region, finish your day by hiking, fishing, boating, camping, or just relaxing in one of two nearby state parks. The beach at Mt. Sunapee State Park is a great place for a swim after

Location
Sullivan County

Endpoints
Newport to Claremont

Mileage
9.8

Roughness Index
2

Surface
Ballast, cinder, sand

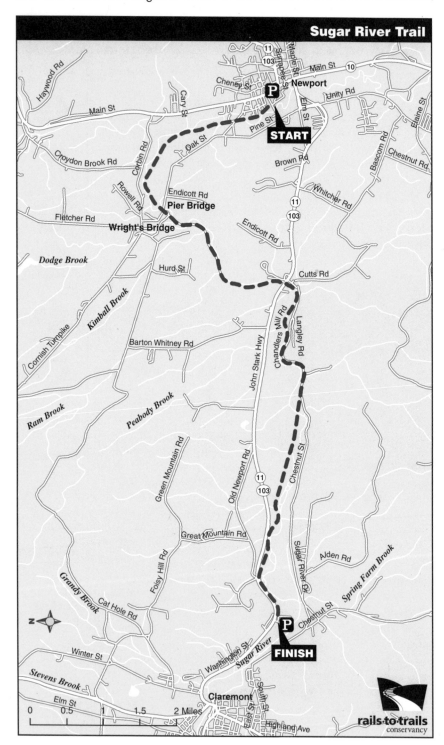

Sugar River Trail

you get off of the trail, and you can take rented kayaks and canoes for a spin on Lake Sunapee. In Washington, Pillsbury State Park offers heavily wooded hiking and mountain biking trails. Seasonal camping is available in both parks. Call for reservations, fees, and hours of operation.

The Sugar River Trail is one of just six rail-trails in New Hampshire that permit motorized use year-round; be prepared to share the trail with ATV users and snowmobilers. Also keep watch for equestrians.

DIRECTIONS

To reach the Newport trailhead, take Interstate 89 to State Route 103 west. In Newport, follow State Route 10 north for a quarter mile past the town green, then turn left on Belknap Avenue. The well-marked trailhead parking lot is on the right.

To reach the Claremont trailhead, follow the above directions to Newport, then follow State Route 11/103 toward Claremont. Where the highway becomes local Washington Street, look for the trailhead parking sign.

Contact: New Hampshire Bureau of Trails
PO Box 1856
Concord, NH 03302
(603) 271-3254
www.nhtrails.org

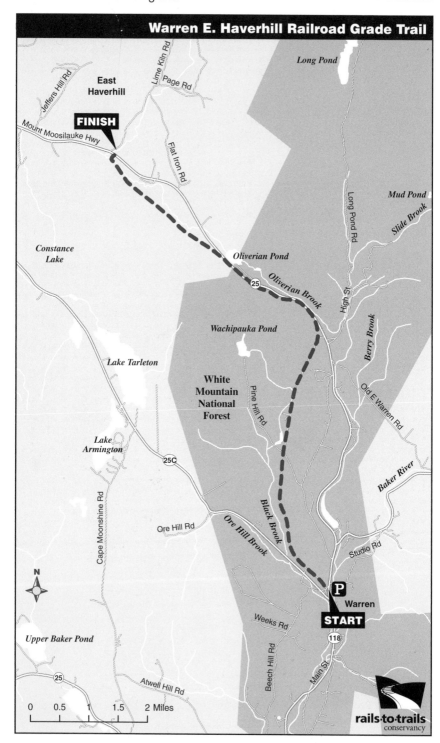

Warren E. Haverhill Railroad Grade Trail

Long Pond

Lime Kiln Rd

Page Rd

Jeffers Hill Rd

East Haverhill

FINISH

Mount Moosilauke Hwy

Flat Iron Rd

Mud Pond

Slide Brook

Long Pond Rd

Constance Lake

Oliverian Pond

25

Oliverian Brook

High St

Berry Brook

Wachipauka Pond

White Mountain National Forest

Lake Tarleton

Pine Hill Rd

Old E Warren Rd

Baker River

Lake Armington

25C

Cape Moonshine Rd

Ore Hill Rd

Ore Hill Brook

Black Brook

Studio Rd

N

P

Warren

START

Weeks Rd

118

Upper Baker Pond

25

Beech Hill Rd

Main St

Atwell Hill Rd

0   0.5   1   1.5   2 Miles

rails·to·trails
conservancy

Warren E. Haverhill Railroad Grade Trail

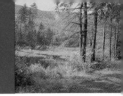

This popular trail starts from an interesting landmark: a Redstone missile brought to Warren by a resident who served in the Army in Alabama in 1970. He found some obsolete missiles in a field and arranged with the Army to transport one back to Warren, aiming to bring something of America's thriving (and far-removed) space program closer to local youth. Placed in the town center in 1971, it remains a prominent fixture.

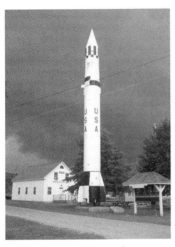

This trailhead has a unique landmark—a Redstone missile.

The rail-trail (a.k.a. the Jesse E. Bushaw Memorial Trail or New Hampshire Snowmobile Corridor No. 5) is a pleasant and picturesque 9.4-mile multipurpose route. The hard-packed dirt surface is generally wide, smooth, and flat, and motorized use is permitted, making it popular among ATV riders in summer and snowmobilers in winter. The trail also welcomes walkers, bikers, equestrians, and anglers eager to try their luck in trailside brooks and ponds.

While most of the route is straight with few technical obstacles, between miles 6 and 7, the trail dips and climbs steeply as it diverges from the railbed to follow State Route 25. Where it rejoins the corridor, the route again runs straight and flat.

Around mile 8, just after you pass the concrete cubes protecting this section of the trail from motorized use, you'll enter the Oliverian Valley Wildlife Preserve's Habitat Management Demonstration Area. Viewing platforms on either side of the path help you keep an eye out for birds and other wildlife.

Location
Grafton County

Endpoints
Warren to East Haverhill

Mileage
9.4

Roughness Index
2

Surface
Dirt

In the final mile, the trail passes under power lines, swings to the right, and crosses a brook. You'll emerge on State Route 25 in East Haverhill between the Oliverian Valley Campground and a baseball field. This trailhead is difficult to find, so begin your journey in Warren.

DIRECTIONS

To reach the Warren trailhead, take Interstate 93 to Exit 26 and follow State Route 25 west about 20 miles to Warren. In Warren, head toward the Redstone missile prominently displayed in the town center. The Warren E. Haverhill Railroad Grade Trail begins along the dirt road that leads into the woods directly behind the missile.

Contact: White Mountain National Forest
Pemigewassett Ranger District
1171 Route 175
Holderness, NH 03245
(603) 536-1315

White Mountains Rail-Trails

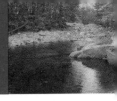

This 18-mile route links the Lincoln Woods, Wilderness, Thoreau Falls, Ethan Pond, and Zealand trails, promising multiday hikes into the pristine White Mountains backcountry. At the midpoint, the nearest road is 7 miles in either direction. That isolation makes for a quiet, reflective walk beside rivers, over hills, and through woods. For most of its length, the route follows the beds of the Lincoln Railroad's East Branch and the Zealand Valley Railroad. Both lines carried lumber out of these mountains from the late 1800s to the early 1900s.

The hike begins atop the steps beside the Lincoln Woods Visitor Center. From here, you'll follow the Lincoln Woods Trail 2.8 miles to the Wilderness Trail. Watch for old railroad ties and logging camp clearings. This stretch used to be part of the Wilderness Trail but was renamed, as it doesn't actually fall within the Pemigewasset Wilderness. You'll encounter many backcountry hikers along this corridor, but the crowds drop off the deeper you venture. The first designated campsite is at the intersection of these two trails.

Location
Grafton County

Endpoints
Within White Mountain National Forest

Mileage
18

Roughness Index
3

Surface
Ballast, gravel, grass, woodchips, dirt, sand

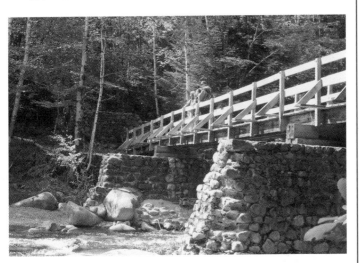

A handful of interconnected rail-trails were built on former logging corridors within the White Mountains.

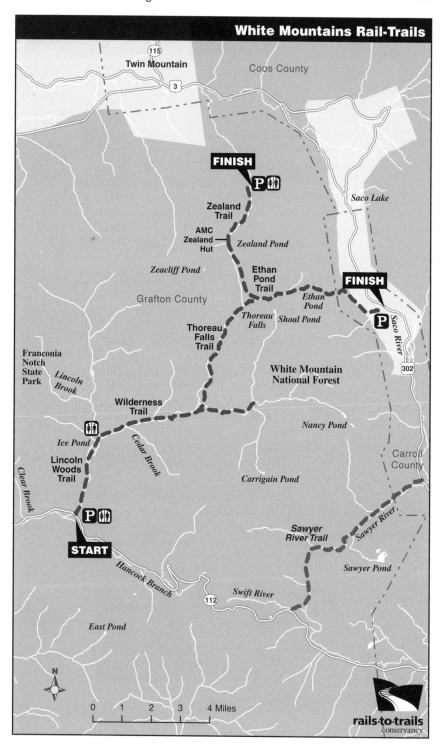

White Mountains Rail-Trails

Twin Mountain

Coos County

115

3

FINISH

Saco Lake

Zealand
Trail

AMC
Zealand
Hut

Zealand Pond

Zeacliff Pond

Ethan
Pond
Trail

Ethan
Pond

FINISH

Grafton County

Thoreau
Falls

Shoal Pond

Saco River

Thoreau
Falls
Trail

White Mountain
National Forest

302

Franconia
Notch
State
Park

Lincoln
Brook

Wilderness
Trail

Cedar Brook

Nancy Pond

Ice Pond

Carroll
County

Lincoln
Woods
Trail

Carrigain Pond

Clear Brook

P

START

Hancock Branch

112

Swift River

Sawyer
River Trail

Sawyer River

Sawyer Pond

East Pond

N

0   1   2   3   4 Miles

rails·to·trails
conservancy

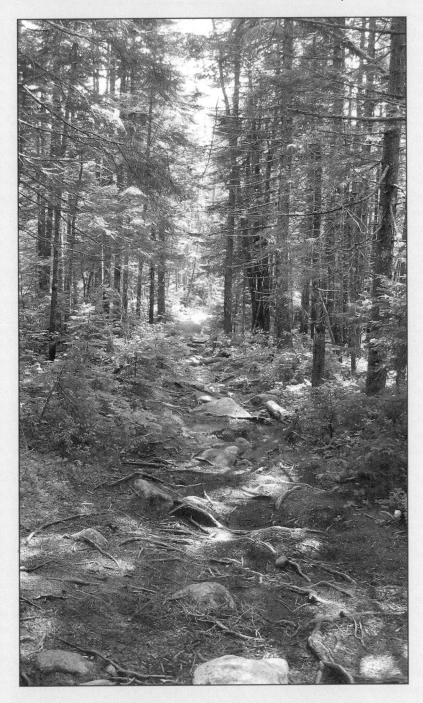

A rugged path cuts through the woods in the White Mountains on one of several rail-trails in the vicinity.

The Wilderness Trail largely keeps to the old railbed. About 4.8 miles from the trailhead, you'll reach a stunning railroad trestle across the East Branch. A half mile farther, the trail crosses a suspension bridge within sight of another dilapidated span, off to the right.

At about 6.2 miles, you'll connect with the Thoreau Falls Trail, which forks to the left. Deviating from the railbed, this trail offers a winding route that rises and plunges amid thick forest along the unspoiled North Fork. The scenic stroll features several interesting stream crossings on old, uneven footbridges, as well as places to stop for a swim. If you do, use caution, as the current can be swift. Follow the trail to the top of Thoreau Falls, find a safe crossing, and pause to enjoy the beautiful mountain views.

The onward route soon meets the bed of the old Zealand Valley Railroad at the Ethan Pond Trail. This corridor encompasses two trails: the Ethan Pond (part of the Appalachian Trail) and the Zealand.

The Ethan Pond Trail keeps to the railbed. Turn left unless you plan to stay at either of two campsites along the right branch to US 302. Leading through a tunnel of trees along the railbed, the left branch soon opens on an outcrop at Zealand Notch, with breathtaking views, of Mt. Bond and other peaks. This is a perfect place to stop for lunch or a rest.

Beyond several rockslides and a series of uneven sections, you'll reach the junction with the Zealand Trail and a spur up to the AMC Zealand Hut. The Zealand continues straight along the railbed, while the spur veers left and climbs steeply 0.2 mile to the hut. Crossing several mountain ponds over wooden footbridges, the Zealand Trail eventually descends to a trailhead parking area on Zealand Road.

DIRECTIONS

To reach the Lincoln Woods trailhead, take Interstate 93 to Exit 32 and follow State Route 112 toward Lincoln. Continue 5.5 miles to the Lincoln Woods parking area. The trailhead is adjacent to the visitor center.

Contact: White Mountain National Forest
Pemigewassett Ranger District
1171 Route 175
Holderness, NH 03245
(603) 536-1315

Windham Depot to Derry Trail

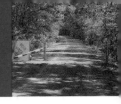

Stretching 4.1 miles north from Windham through woodlands to Derry, the trail runs on the same former rail bed network on which the Rockingham Recreational Trail (see page 159) is built. Part of a planned 29-mile rail-trail system that will go from Salem, New Hampshire, on the Massachusetts border to the state capital in Concord.

This section of trail, which extends from the Windham Rail Trail, begins 600 feet north of the restored Windham Depot. Except for a short, paved stretch in Derry, the surface is gravel, cinder, and sand. The corridor passes through deciduous woods, wetlands, and swamps. Beaver activity is responsible for some of the wetlands, and you might spot a beaver lodge or perhaps a beaver itself at work on a dam.

Near its midpoint, the trail passes beneath a road through a narrow culvert with low overhead clearance; cyclists may want to dismount and walk through. To avoid the culvert altogether, follow the well-worn path up to the road and carefully cross to the other side to pick up the rail-trail.

Location
Rockingham County

Endpoints
Windham to Derry

Mileage
4.1

Roughness Index
2

Surface
Asphalt, gravel, cinder, sand

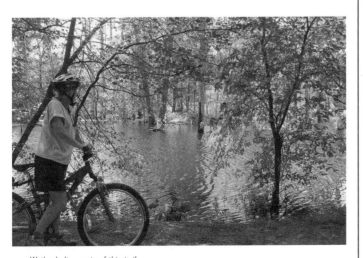
Wetlands line parts of this trail.

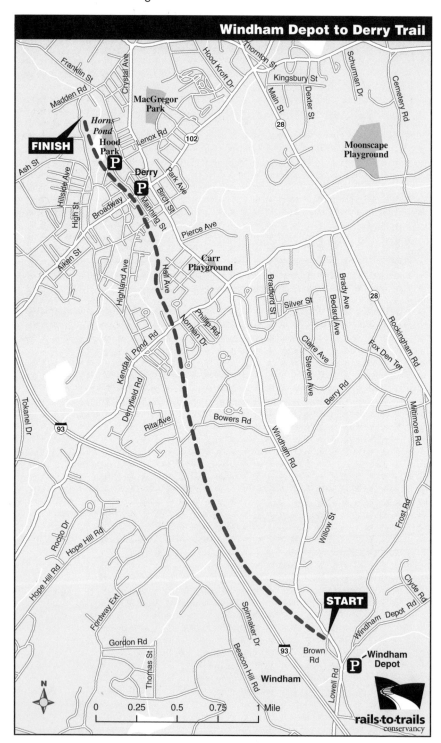

Windham Depot to Derry Trail

Approaching Derry, the surface changes to asphalt. The town hosts two of America's oldest private schools: Pinkerton Academy, founded in 1814 and still operating, and the defunct 1824 Adams Female Seminary. Another claim to fame: Astronaut Alan Shepard, the first American in space, was born and raised in Derry. A restored train depot now houses a restaurant with outdoor seating. Consider pausing for a break here or at one of Derry's other eateries.

Back on the trail, you'll soon cross State Route 102. Here, the trail temporarily leaves the old rail bed on a pathway marked by red brick pavers. North of town, Hood Park signals the trail's end, though the right-of-way continues several hundred feet beyond Hood Park, before it dead-ends at a residential complex.

DIRECTIONS

To reach the trailhead in Windham, take Interstate 93 to Exit 3 and head west on State Route 111 toward Windham. After about a mile, turn right on North Lowell Road. Just beyond the interstate underpass, North Lowell intersects with Windham Depot Road, where you bear right. Park at the restored Windham Depot, about 150 yards up on the right.

To reach the Hood Park trailhead in Derry, take I-93 to Exit 4 and head east on State Route 102. In town, turn left on Manning Street, which ends at the Hood Park trailhead. Parking is available.

Contact: New Hampshire Bureau of Trails
PO Box 856
Concord, NH 03302
(603) 271-3254
www.nhtrails.org

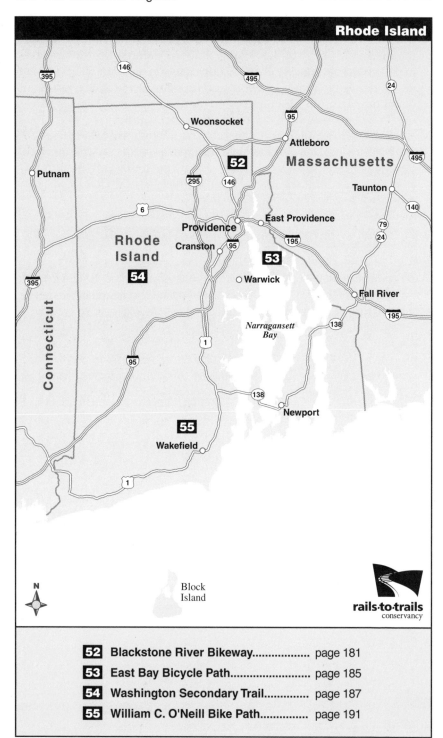

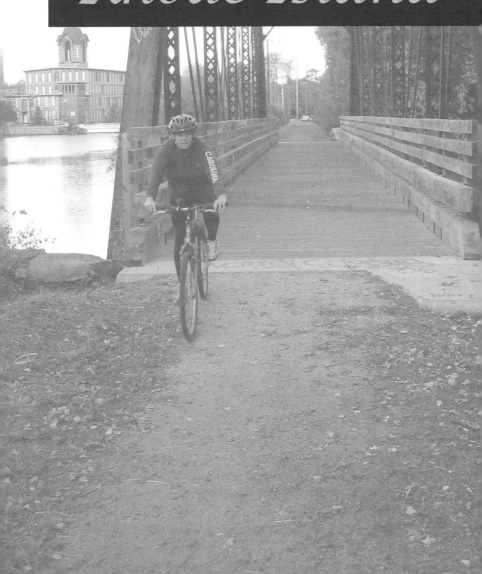

Rhode Island

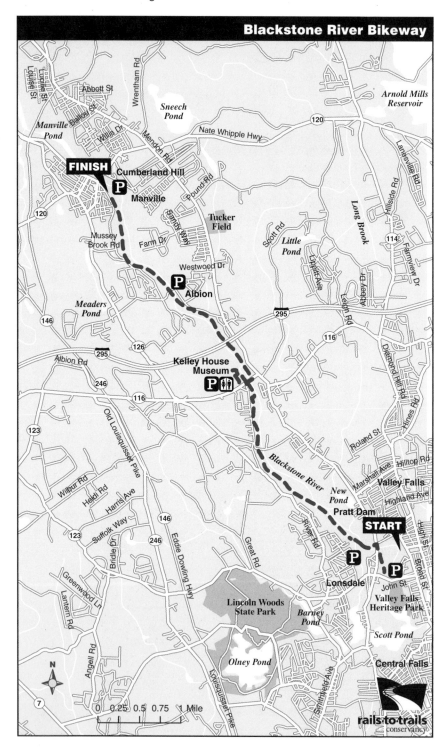

Blackstone River Bikeway

Blackstone River Bikeway

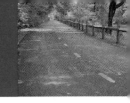

T he Blackstone River Bikeway represents a big undertaking in this tiny state: The 6.8-mile trail is the largest open segment on a nearly 50-mile former rail corridor that will eventually connect Providence to Worcester, Massachusetts.

A restored drive-in movie theater sign "featuring" the Blackstone River Bikeway greets you at the trail's current south end on John Street in Lonsdale. From the start, you'll be treated to many picturesque scenes of the wide, churning Blackstone River and the placid, historic canal. After a mile, you'll cross over the Pratt Dam on the a six-span bridge, which sits atop the original railroad piers and abutment.

Beyond the dam, the bikeway turns right and continues north (the path leading straight ends at a parking lot). Note: You may run into construction at the Martin Street road bridge, which has temporarily divided the trail into two segments.

Northbound toward the village of Ashton, the trail alternately follows and parallels the historic canal towpath. Keep an eye out for a large brick textile mill; the

Location
Providence County

Endpoints
Lonsdale to
Manville

Mileage
6.8

**Roughness
Index**
1

Surface
Asphalt

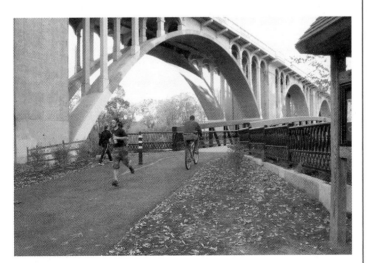

The trail crosses the Blackstone River, for which it is named.

canal was built to transport cotton goods from the mill to Worcester and Providence in the 1800s.

Ashton marks the approximate trail midpoint. You could begin or end your journey here by parking on Route 116 or at the visitor center along Interstate 295, which provides restrooms and information. Each parking lot offers a connecting spur on a slight incline to the trail.

History buffs may choose to visit the historic Kelley House Museum, former home of Wilbur Kelley, a ship captain and mill owner. Nestled between the river and canal, the museum relates the transportation and industrial history of each waterway.

Continuing north, the trail parallels the active Providence & Worcester Railroad all the way to the end, even sharing a bridge across the river in Albion. The building materials for this stretch of the rail-trail were shipped by and unloaded right off the train.

While the trail currently ends in Manville, sections continuing north are under construction.

DIRECTIONS

To reach the Lonsdale trailhead, take Interstate 295 to State Route 146 south. Exit onto State Route 123 east and follow it to John Street. Look for the restored drive-in movie theater sign that marks the trailhead.

To reach the Manville trailhead, also take I-295 to Route 146 south and exit onto Route 123 east. Turn left on Route 122 north toward Manville. In town, turn left on Manville Hill Road, cross the river, then turn left on Main Street. You'll see the trail on the left. Turn left, downhill, and cross the railroad tracks and the trail to reach the parking lot.

Contact: Rhode Island Division of Parks & Recreation
2321 Hartford Avenue
Johnston, RI 02919
(401) 222-2632
www.riparks.com

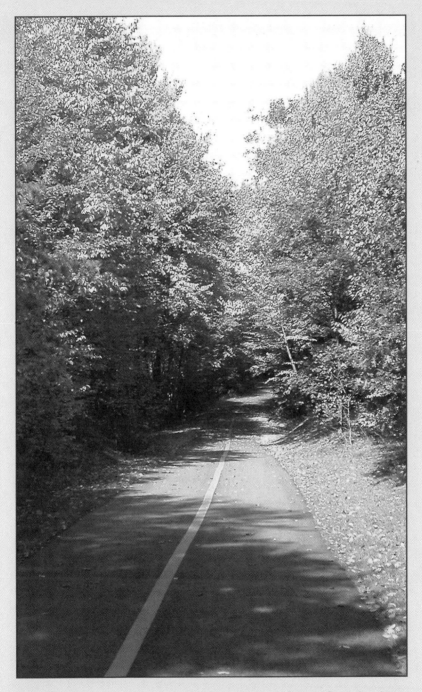

The Blackstone River Bikeway cuts through forested areas, often between the Blackstone River and an adjacent canal.

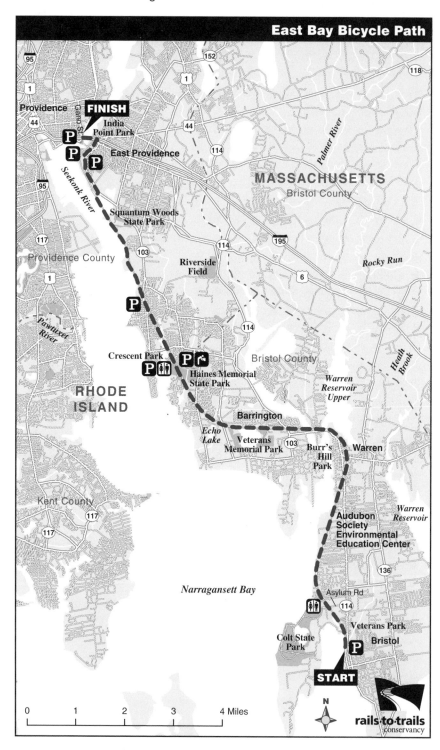

East Bay Bicycle Path

East Bay Bicycle Path

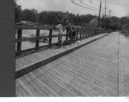

Rhode Island's best-known rail-trail, the East Bay Bicycle Path, hugs the shores of Narragansett Bay, from Bristol in the south, north to India Point Park in Providence. The 14-mile paved path accommodates a wide variety of uses. Markers on the pavement every half mile help you keep track of your progress.

The trail takes you through an alternating landscape of stunning natural areas, as well as more urban enclaves. Spur trails lead to several parks and conservation areas, including Colt State Park in Bristol, Burr's Hill Park in Warren, and Veterans Memorial Park and Haines Memorial State Park in Barrington.

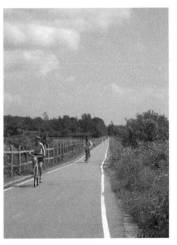

This smooth trail allows you to glide through several natural areas.

In Bristol, watch for an intersection on the path marked by bike racks. Here, a path leads to the Rhode Island Audubon Society's Environmental Education Center. The center features a state-of-the art, fully accessible natural history museum and aquarium, as well as all-season guided tours, nature walks, and special family programs.

Approaching Providence, you'll cross the Interstate 195 bridge to India Point Park, the path's northern terminus. The park, built on the rail bed and scrap metal yards in 1974, was originally a port for trading ships bound for the East and West Indies in the 1700s. After 1850, with the arrival of the rail line, it became a debarkation point for new immigrants to America. Train service on this route operated from 1855 until 1974. In 1900, the New Haven Railroad, which owned the line at the time, converted it to electric car service using overhead lines.

Location
Bristol County

Endpoints
Independence Park in Bristol to India Point park in Providence

Mileage
14

Roughness Index
1

Surface
Asphalt

A half-mile detour from the trail in Riverside leads to Crescent Park and the Looff Carousel. To get to the park, head east on Crescent View Avenue where it intersects the trail. A sculptural masterpiece of wood, the carousel features 62 exquisitely carved figures and four chariots. Dating to 1895, it's listed on the National Register of Historic Places.

DIRECTIONS

To reach the Colt State Park trailhead in Bristol, take Interstate 195 to State Route 114 south toward Bristol. In Bristol, turn right on Asylum Road.

To reach the Providence trailhead, take Interstate 95 to I-195 east to the Gano Street exit. Turn left into India Point Park. The trailhead is on the right; ramps lead up to the bridge where the path begins as a separated corridor alongside traffic.

There are many other places to park along the trail. The closest parking lots to the northern terminus are on Veterans Memorial Parkway in East Providence. Traveling east on I-195 from Providence, take the Riverside exit. You'll find two parking lots on the right.

Contact: Colt State Park
Bristol, RI 02809
(401) 253-7482
www.riparks.com/eastbay.htm

Washington Secondary Trail

The Washington Secondary Trail (a.k.a. Cranston–Warwick Bike Path) actually comprises four completed, but not yet connected trails along an old Hartford, Providence, & Fishkill Railroad corridor. Together, the Cranston Bikeway, Warwick Bike Path, West Warwick Greenway, and Coventry Greenway create 12.7 miles of open trail. When completed, the overall trail will run 25 miles from Providence to the Moosup Valley State Park Trail in Connecticut.

The rail line was used primarily to carry goods to manufacturers, lumberyards, grain distributors, and the old Narragansett Brewery in Cranston. From the path, you'll see evidence of mills the freight cars once serviced.

The first 10 miles of continuous trail begin at Depot Street in Cranston. You'll start out on the Cranston Bikeway, a neighborhood trail that passes through commercial and residential areas before reaching a quiet, wooded section flanked by split-rail fencing. Before leaving Cranston, you will pass through Oaklawn Village Center, with a parking lot and gazebo, and cross Meshanticut Brook.

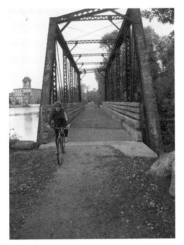

From the trail, you can view old mill buildings that dot the banks of the Pawtuxet River.

Location
Providence and Kent counties

Endpoints
Cranston to Coventry

Mileage
12.7

Roughness Index
1

Surface
Asphalt

The trail then takes a quick, 1.5-mile spin through Warwick on the Warwick Bikepath and into West Warwick. Along this section, the route negotiates two curves, quite unusual for a rail-trail.

At West Warwick, the trail becomes known locally as the West Warwick Greenway. You'll travel through an old mill area along the Pawtuxet River. This area is a center of redevelopment activity, with conversions of

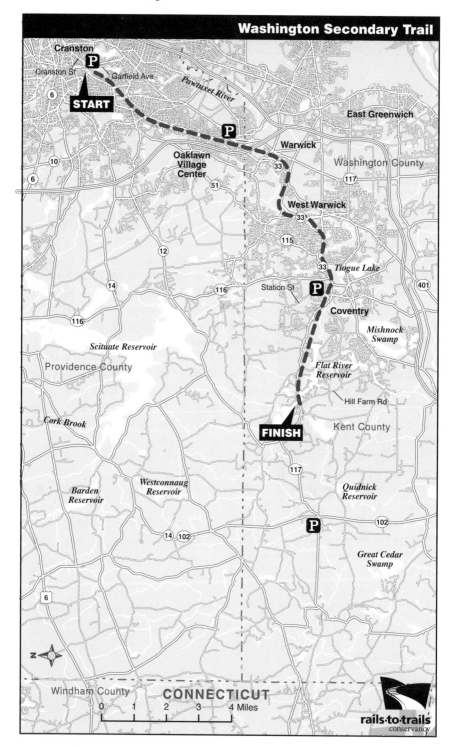

Washington Secondary Trail

Cranston

Cranston St

Garfield Ave

Pawtuxet River

START

6

10

6

Oaklawn
Village
Center

51

12

14

116

116

Scituate Reservoir

Providence County

Cork Brook

Barden
Reservoir

Westconnaug
Reservoir

14 102

6

33

Warwick

East Greenwich

Washington County

117

West Warwick

33

115

33 Tiogue Lake

401

116

Station St

Coventry

Mishnock
Swamp

Flat River
Reservoir

Hill Farm Rd

FINISH

Kent County

117

Quidnick
Reservoir

102

Great Cedar
Swamp

Windham County   **CONNECTICUT**

0   1   2   3   4 Miles

rails·to·trails
conservancy

old mill buildings. A red New York, New Haven, & Hartford Railroad caboose stands proudly by the trail.

Soon after the village of Arctic, the West Warwick Greenway ends at the Coventry town line, where a 2.3-mile gap is currently being developed as a trail.

To reach the next section of open trail, head west along Route 117 to Station Street in Coventry. Here, you can hop on the Coventry Greenway for a peaceful 2.7-mile trek through a rural, wooded area with views of the Flat River Reservoir. The trail surface is paved right up to trail's end near Hill Farm Road. Eventually, this section will link with the Trestle Trail (still under development) and extend the Washington Secondary Trail straight through to Connecticut.

DIRECTIONS

To reach the Cranston trailhead, take Interstate 95 to Exit 16 and follow State Route 10 north. Take the Cranston Street/Niantic Avenue exit and turn left at the bottom of the exit onto Niantic Avenue. At the light, turn left on Cranston Street. At the next light, turn left on Garfield Avenue and look for the Lowe's on the right at Cranston Parkade. The trailhead and parking area are behind Lowe's.

To reach trailhead parking in Coventry, take I-95 to Exit 10 and head west on Route 117 toward Coventry. The trail parallels 117 as you enter town. Just past the firehouse, turn right on Station Street. The parking lot is on the left.

Contact: Town of Coventry Parks & Recreation
1670 Flat River Road
Coventry, RI 02816
(401) 822-9107

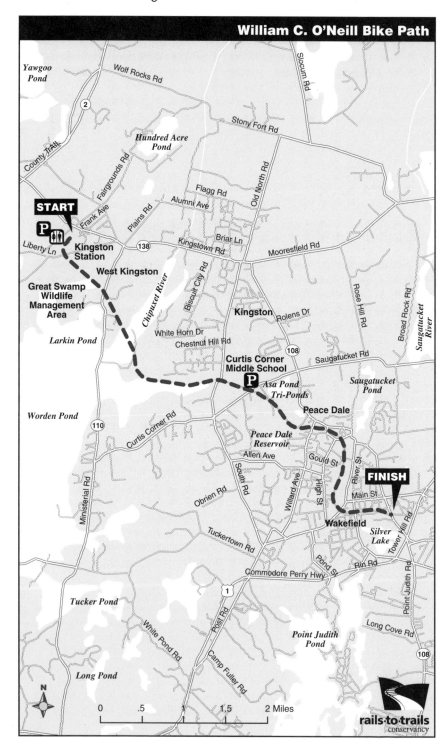

William C. O'Neill Bike Path

Yawgoo Pond

Wolf Rocks Rd

Slocum Rd

2

County TRAIL

Hundred Acre Pond

Stony Fort Rd

Old North Rd

Flagg Rd

Alumni Ave

Fairgrounds Rd

Plains Rd

Frank Ave

START

P

Liberty Ln

Kingston Station

138

Kingstown Rd

Briar Ln

Mooresfield Rd

Rose Hill Rd

Broad Rock Rd

Saugatucket River

West Kingston

Biscuit City Rd

Chipuxet River

Great Swamp Wildlife Management Area

Larkin Pond

White Horn Dr

Chestnut Hill Rd

Kingston

Rolens Dr

108

Saugatucket Rd

Curtis Corner Middle School

P

Asa Pond Tri-Ponds

Saugatucket Pond

Peace Dale

Worden Pond

110

Curtis Corner Rd

Peace Dale Reservoir

Allen Ave

Gould St

River St

FINISH

Ministerial Rd

South Rd

Willard Ave

High St

Main St

Obrien Rd

Wakefield

Silver Lake

Tower Hill Rd

Tuckertown Rd

Pond St

Rin Rd

Point Judith Rd

Commodore Perry Hwy

1

Tucker Pond

White Pond Rd

Post Rd

Camp Fuller Rd

Point Judith Pond

Long Cove Rd

108

Long Pond

N

0   .5   1   1.5   2 Miles

rails·to·trails
conservancy

William C. O'Neill Bike Path

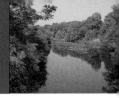

Named for the late state senator who spearheaded development of the trail, the William C. O'Neill Bike Path (a.k.a. South County Bike Path) follows the route of the former Narragansett Pier Railroad, which connected the coastal village of South Kingston with the Narragansett Pier. Built in 1876, the railroad carried passengers to the pier, where they caught the ferry to Newport. It also delivered coal and lumber from the bay to inland villages. In 1921, rail buses—actual buses adapted to ride the rails—replaced regular passenger cars on the line. Locals affectionately called these unique buses Mickey-Dinks, after two of the drivers.

Starting from the newly restored Kingston Station (home to the Rhode Island Railroad Museum; open weekends), this 6.1-mile bike path traverses the Great Swamp Wildlife Management Area. Particularly in the spring and fall, you'll encounter flocks of migratory birds. Just beyond Curtis Corner Middle School, footpaths on either side of the trail lead to Tri-Ponds Park, which features three ponds, streams, 2 miles of nature trails, resident wildlife, and a nature center. Continuing on the bike path, you'll wind through the quaint towns

Location
Washington County

Endpoints
West Kingston to Wakefield

Mileage
6.1

Roughness Index
1

Surface
Asphalt

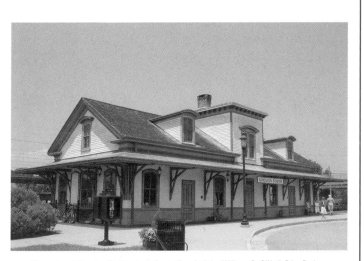

The restored Kingston Station is at the trailhead of the William C. O'Neill Bike Path.

191

of Peace Dale and Wakefield, both rich in historical landmarks. The path abruptly ends at Kingstown Road.

Plans are underway to extend the trail another 2 miles to the ocean. Until then, if you want to travel to the beach, turn right at the end of the bike path onto Kingstown Road and follow it through the rotary all the way to its end. The ocean is straight ahead; Narragansett Pier is on the left. Stop in at a restaurant along the water to savor ocean views and sample the Ocean State's famous quahogs, clam cakes, and Rhode Island clam chowder.

DIRECTIONS

Kingston Station is accessible by car, train, and bus.

By car from Providence, take Interstate 95 south to Exit 9 and follow State Route 4 south to US Hwy. 1 south. From US 1, head west about 7 miles on Route 138, which becomes Mooresfield Road, then Kingstown Road. Turn left on Railroad Avenue into the station. The trail begins at the south end of the main parking lot.

The station is an active stop on Amtrak's Northeast line between Boston and Washington, DC. RIPTA (Rhode Island Public Transportation Authority) buses also serve the station.

There is no parking at the Wakefield terminus, but parking is available at Curtis Corner Middle School in Peace Dale. From Kingstown Road, follow Route 108 south into town and turn right on Curtis Corner Road. The school is at 301 Curtis Corner.

Contact: Friends of William C. O'Neill Bike Path
481 Post Road
Wakefield, RI 02879
(401) 783-8886

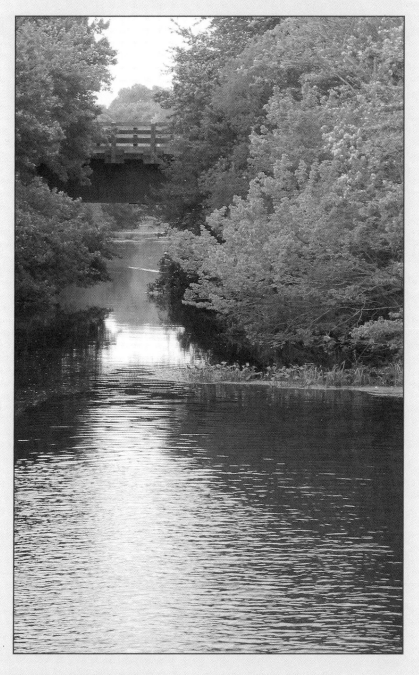

Rhode Island's William C. O'Neill Bike Path was named for the late state senator who championed the trail. Streams and ponds along the route already provide a peaceful setting, and plans are being made to extend it to the ocean.

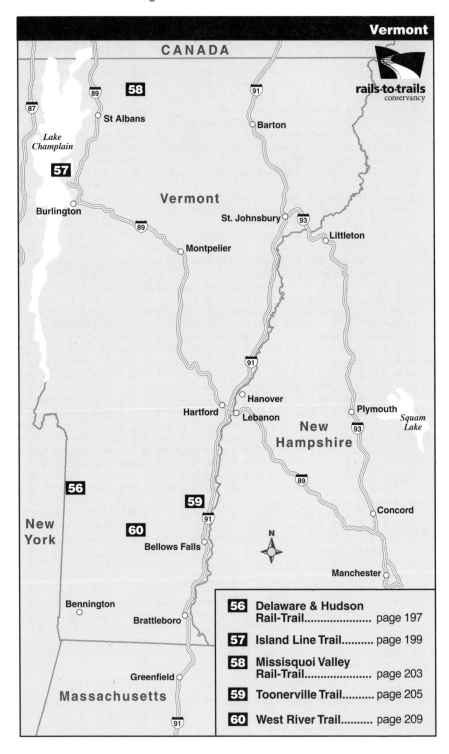

Vermont

rails-to-trails
conservancy

CANADA

58

St Albans

Barton

Lake Champlain

57

Vermont

Burlington

St. Johnsbury

Littleton

Montpelier

Hanover

Hartford   Lebanon

Plymouth

Squam Lake

New Hampshire

56

New York

59

60

Concord

Bellows Falls

Manchester

N

Bennington

Brattleboro

Greenfield

Massachusetts

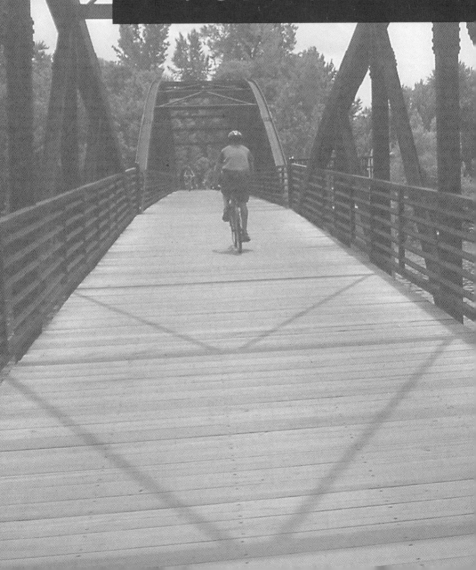

Vermont

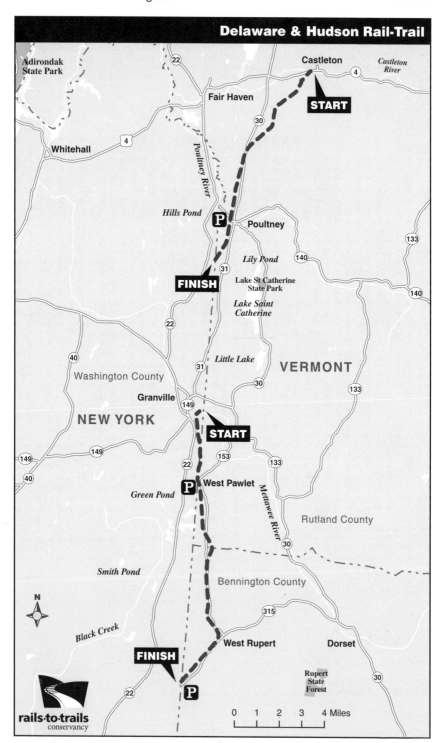

Delaware & Hudson Rail-Trail

Delaware & Hudson Rail-Trail

While hugging the New York state line, the Delaware & Hudson Rail-Trail quietly rambles over the rolling hills and farmland of western Vermont. The 22.3-mile D&H actually comprises two trails split in nearly equal sections, each providing quintessential Vermont solitude.

The trail traces an old Delaware & Hudson line that operated between Rutland and Albany, New York, playing a vital role in the slate industry in the late 1800s and early 1900s. Where the right-of-way crosses the border into New York, the corridor has not been developed as a trail, hence the gap.

To explore the northern section, begin at the Castleton trailhead. From the campus of Castleton State College, the trail delves into lush pockets of northern hardwood trees and provides a glimpse of Vermont farmland. Seven miles along, you'll reach Poultney, where a temporary detour veers from the defined corridor onto the town's sleepy, downtown streets. Rejoining the trail on the south end of town, you'll continue another 2.5 miles before ending abruptly at the New York state line, where a sign marks the end of the trial.

Location
Rutland and Bennington counties

Endpoints
Castleton to West Rupert

Mileage
22.3

Roughness Index
2

Surface
Ballast, gravel, sand

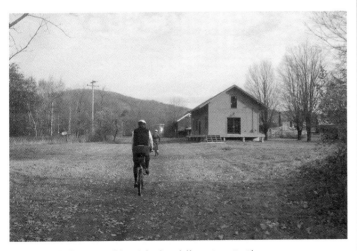

This trail offers a peaceful meander through Vermont countryside.

197

The southern section of the trail begins at the state line just north of West Pawlet. The best spot to access the trail is at the West Pawlet trailhead, which is approximately 2.5 miles south of the northern terminus. This 2.5-mile stretch into town is densely forested and ends at trailhead parking near an industrial site. South of town, the trail opens up a bit, offering sweeping views of the surrounding hills and countryside. Don't be surprised to see deer all along this trail. After passing a parking area outside the small village of West Rupert, the trail continues only a half mile farther before reaching its southern terminus, ending at the state border.

DIRECTIONS

Northern Section: To reach the Castleton trailhead from Rutland, take US Route 4 west to Exit 5, head west a half mile on State Route 4A, and turn left into the entrance of Castleton State College on Seminary Street. Turn right into the visitor parking area. At the end of the lot are rows of designated trail parking spaces.

To reach the Poultney trailhead from Rutland, take US 7 south to Wallingford, then head west on Route 140 into Poultney. In town, turn left on Grove Street, then right on Bentley Street. The trailhead is on the left.

Southern Section: To access the West Pawlet trailhead from Rutland, take US 4 west to Exit 4, head south on Route 30 about 9 miles, then turn south on Route 153 into West Pawlet. At the T-junction with Egg Street, turn right. The trailhead is on the right.

To reach the West Rupert trailhead, follow State Route 153 south to the village of West Rupert. Make a right turn on Hebron Road, and follow it until you see the trail.

Contact: Vermont Department of Forests, Parks, & Recreation
271 North Main Street, Suite 215
Rutland, VT 05701
(802) 786-3857
www.vtfpr.org

Island Line Trail

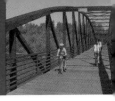

One of New England's most visited and spectacular rail-trails, the paved, 12-mile Island Line Trail (formerly known as the Burlington Bikeway) skirts the waterfront in the hip college town of Burlington, strings together a series of shoreline parks, and offers spectacular views of Lake Champlain and New York's Adirondack Mountains. Best of all, the relatively flat trail features a unique and scenic trip out over the lake on a marble causeway.

The trail's official start point is at the Oakledge Park

trailhead on Flynn Street in south Burlington, which offers plenty of parking and amenities. The route leads north along the waterfront. At 2.1 miles, you'll reach the Union Station trailhead on King Street. (If you opt to begin here, bring extra change for the parking meters.)

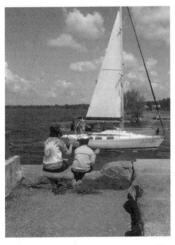

Burlington's waterfront is characterized by ferries, sailboats, and the Island Line Trail.

Pause to admire lake views at the public North Beach Park trailhead at mile 3.4. A seasonal snack bar serves a variety of food and beverages.

At mile 5.1, you'll enter Leddy Park in Burlington's New North End. The city's largest park, Leddy provides full amenities, parking, a sandy beach, a picnic area with tables and grills, and more lakefront vistas.

A few miles north, you'll reach the Winooski River Bridge. This beautiful span—and the associated half-mile elevated boardwalk across the Delta Park floodplain—is the crucial link that united the Burlington Bikeway and Colchester Causeway rail-trails in 2004, after 15 years of planning.

Location
Chittenden County

Endpoints
Burlington to Colchester Causeway

Mileage
12.1

Roughness Index
1

Surface
Asphalt, crushed stone

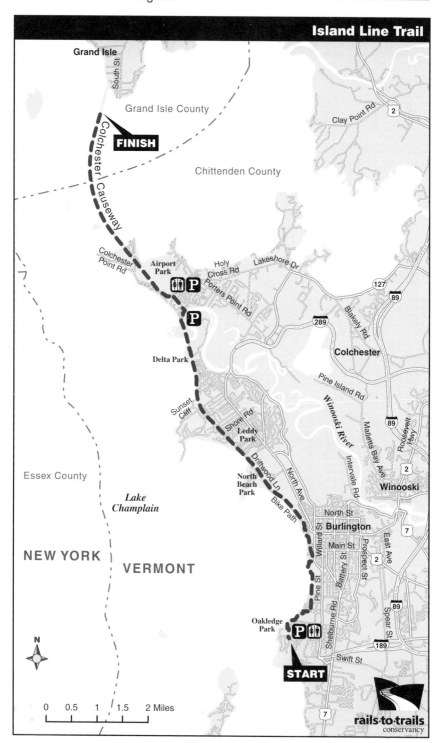

Island Line Trail

Grand Isle

South St

Grand Isle County

Clay Point Rd

2

Colchester Causeway

FINISH

Chittenden County

Colchester Point Rd

Airport Park

Holy Cross Rd

Lakeshore Dr

127

89

Porters Point Rd

289

Blakely Rd

Delta Park

Colchester

Pine Island Rd

89

Sunset Cliff

Shore Rd

Leddy Park

Winooski River

Malletts Bay Ave

Roosevelt Hwy

North Beach Park

Driftwood Ln

North Ave

Bike Path

Intervale Rd

2

Winooski

Lake Champlain

North St

Willard St

Burlington

Prospect St

East Ave

7

NEW YORK

VERMONT

Essex County

Main St

Battery St

2

Pine St

89

Spear St

Oakledge Park

Shelburne Rd

189

START

Swift St

N

0   0.5   1   1.5   2 Miles

7

rails·to·trails
conservancy

The causeway itself lies farther north, just beyond Colchester's residential neighborhoods and Airport Park. Built in 1900 atop huge marble boulders, the 2.5-mile raised railbed slices across Lake Champlain for unparalleled views. As you sail along the crushed stone surface, you'll have a sense of skimming the water's surface. The causeway ends abruptly out on the lake, where a seasonal bike ferry connects with South Hero.

DIRECTIONS

To reach the Oakledge Park trailhead in Burlington, take Interstate 89 to Exit 13 and follow I-189 south to US 7. Turn right on US Route 7 north, then left on Flynn Avenue. Follow Flynn to its end and look for signs to Oakledge Park.

To reach the Airport Park trailhead in Colchester, take Interstate 89 to Exit 17 (US Route 2). Follow signs for US Route 2/US 7/ Lake Champlain Islands/Colchester. Turn right onto Theodore Roosevelt Hwy./Route 2. Continue for 3 miles before turning right on Bay Road, and then take another right onto West Lakeshore Drive. West Lakeshore becomes Holy Cross Road and then Colchester Point Road. Trail parking is on the right at Airport Park on Colchester Point Road.

Contact: Local Motion
1 Steele Street, #103
Burlington, VT 05401
(802) 652-2453
www.localmotion.org

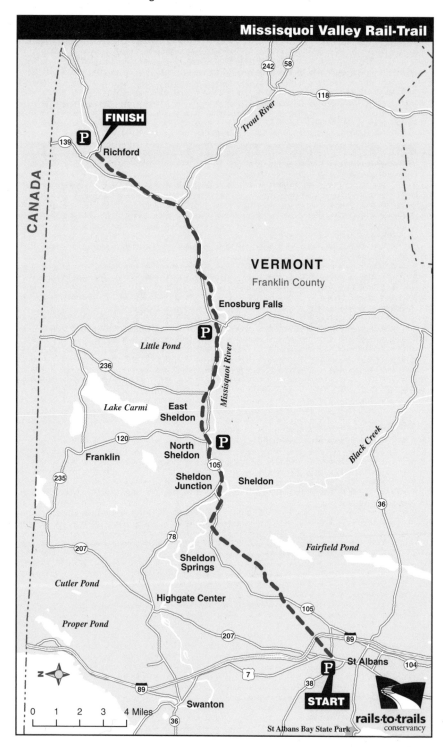

Missisquoi Valley Rail-Trail

Missisquoi Valley Rail-Trail

Winding northeast from St. Albans to Richford, just south of the Vermont/Québec border, the Missisquoi Valley Rail-Trail affords visitors direct access to northwest Vermont dairy country. In winter, hardy users take to the 26.1-mile route on snowshoes, cross-country skis, and snowmobiles.

Tracing the bed of the Richford Branch of the Central Vermont Railway, the corridor never exceeds a 3 percent grade. The gentle terrain makes this a family-friendly ride and the perfect venue for enjoying postcard images of rural farms, forests, and fields.

The well-groomed, crushed limestone trail begins in St. Albans, which hosts a good selection of restaurants, as well as a museum with railroad memorabilia. The first 10 miles run along State Route 105 past rolling farmland, woods, and a wetland area. Reaching the banks of the Missisquoi River, you'll cross an old railroad trestle into Sheldon Junction, a rural town offering more restaurants and restroom facilities.

Linking the communities of North Sheldon and South Franklin, the onward trail skirts the river past expansive cornfields and picturesque dairy farms.

Location
Franklin County

Endpoints
St. Albans to
Richford

Mileage
26.1

**Roughness
Index**
2

Surface
Crushed stone

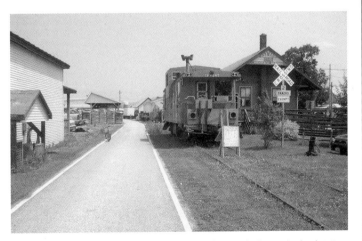

The Missisquoi Valley Rail-Trail showcases a red caboose and a historical railroad station at its Enosburg Falls trailhead.

The next main trailhead is in Enosburg Falls. Look for the vintage red caboose alongside the old railroad station at the side of the trail. Beside the station is an interesting little museum with memorabilia from the past two centuries, offering historical glimpses of the town that once dubbed itself the "Dairy Center of the World."

After Enosburg Falls, as you near the eastern terminus in Richford, the trail meanders through more quintessential Vermont countryside, with occasional glimpses of the Missisquoi River. The trail and river eventually part ways at an old trestle 3 miles shy of the trail's end in town.

DIRECTIONS

To reach the St. Albans trailhead, take Interstate 89 to Exit 20 and follow US Route 7 south to State Route 105/Sheldon Road. Turn left on 105 and drive one block to the trailhead.

To reach the Richford trailhead, continue north on Route 105 into downtown Richford, turn right on Troy Street, and follow Troy until you see the trailhead on the right.

Contact: Northeast Regional Planning Commission
155 Lake Street
St. Albans, VT 05478
(802) 524-5959

Toonerville Trail

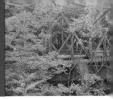

T he Toonerville Trail (a.k.a. Springfield Greenway) spans 3 meticulously maintained miles from the downtown business district of Springfield southeast to the western bank of the Connecticut River at the Vermont/New Hampshire border. The Springfield Terminal Railway once operated an electric rail line connecting Springfield to Charlestown, New Hampshire, across the state boarder. The trolley, affectionately nicknamed the "Toonerville Trolley" after a popular cartoon strip that ran until 1947. Established in the 1890s, it was Vermont's longest surviving passenger trolley service.

The paved trail begins at the Robert B. Jones Industrial Center, just east of downtown. Starting your trip here is a breeze: There's plenty of parking, the trailhead is easy to find, and the first 2 miles of the trail follow a gentle downhill grade along the Black River. A tributary of the Connecticut, the Black River powered mills in the 18th and 19th centuries, although today you're more likely to spot a kingfisher or blue heron than evidence of the mills.

At mile 1.5, the trail spans the Black River by way of a rustic former trolley bridge. Before crossing, venture

Location
Windsor County

Endpoints
Springfield, VT, to
Charlestown, NH

Mileage
3.1

**Roughness
Index**
1

Surface
Asphalt

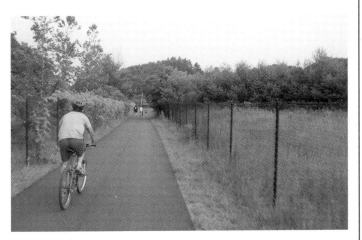

Built on a former trolley line, the Toonerville Trail's well-groomed path makes for an easy trip.

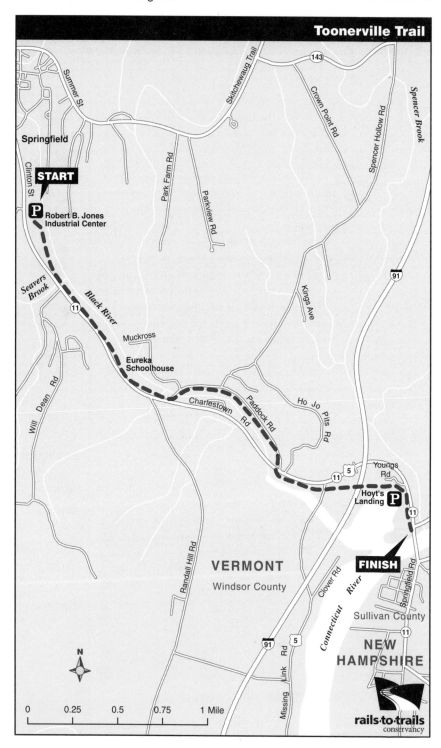

off-trail for a visit to the 1795 Eureka Schoolhouse. It is the state's oldest one-room school. In the 1960s, crews moved the building to its present location and restored it. Open from May to October, it now serves as a tourist information center.

Beyond the bridge, the trail takes a short detour on quiet Paddock Road before rejoining the corridor and passing beneath US Route 11. The Toonerville Trail continues for another half mile before reaching a parking area for Hoyt's Landing at the confluence of the rivers, a popular spot for fishing, swimming, and canoeing. Beyond the landing, the trail crosses beneath US 11 once more, ending a third of a mile later at US Route 5.

DIRECTIONS

To reach the Springfield trailhead, take Interstate 91 to Exit 7 and follow US Route 11 north toward Springfield for approximately 2.5 miles. Watch for the Robert B. Jones Industrial Center on the right. There is ample parking here.

To reach the Hoyt's Landing trailhead from I-91, take Exit 7 and follow US 11 toward Charlestown, News Hampshire. Hoyt's Landing, and trail parking, is on the right.

Contact: Springfield Parks & Recreation
96 Main Street
Springfield, VT 05156
(802) 885-2727
www.springfieldvt.com/toonerville.htm

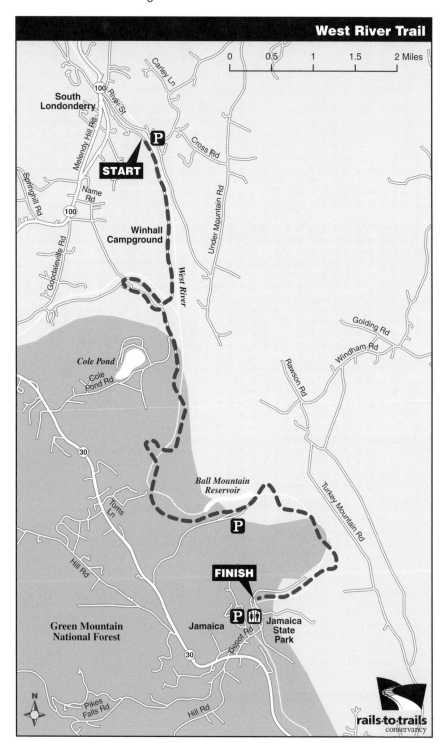

0   0.5   1   1.5   2 Miles

South
Londonderry

Carley Ln

River St

100

Melendy Hill Rd

P

START

Cross Rd

Under Mountain Rd

Name
Rd

100

Winhall
Campground

West River

Springhill Rd

Goodaleville Rd

Cole Pond

Cole
Pond Rd

Golding Rd

Windham Rd

Rawson Rd

30

Ball Mountain
Reservoir

P

Toms
Ln

Turkey Mountain Rd

Hill Rd

FINISH

P 🚻

Green Mountain
National Forest

Jamaica

Depot Rd

Jamaica
State
Park

30

N

Pikes
Falls Rd

Hill Rd

rails·to·trails
conservancy

West River Trail

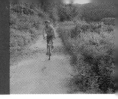

Following the floodplain of the West River Valley, the 12.5-mile West River Trail (a.k.a. Railroad Bed Trail) appeals to a wide range of trail users. The rail-trail has a nearly level surface, ideal for walkers, cyclists, and equestrians, while a rugged section satisfies avid hikers. The West River Railroad once traveled this corridor, linking the industrial communities of Brattleboro and Londonderry.

Starting in South Londonderry, the trail takes you for a scenic 2.7-mile tour along the gently flowing river before reaching the Winhall Campground. Suitable for all trail uses, this section really captures the essence of this quiet river valley. Once you reach the campground, there is a gap in the trail. Follow the campground roads up to the bridge where you can safely cross a small creek, then follow the campground roads back down again to rejoin the trail along the river bank, where you can continue on the rail-trail.

A half mile past the campground, the trail seems to reach an abrupt end. Mountain bikers will want to turn back here. But if you're up for a rugged hike, look to

Location
Windham County

Endpoints
South Londonderry to Jamaica State Park

Mileage
12.5

Roughness Index
2

Surface
Gravel, sand

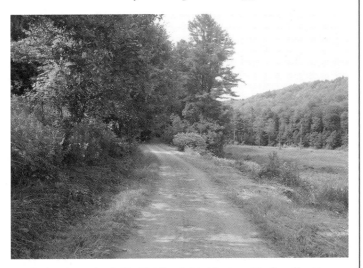

It takes some work to find the West River Trail, but the views of the Green Mountains are well worth it.

your right for the purple marker indicating the continuation of the trail.

The rail-trail continues for 3.5 miles before reaching the massive Ball Mountain Dam. Follow the trail signs closely for a route to the top of the dam, and you'll be treated to spectacular views of the river valley flanked by the gentle slopes of the Green Mountains. On the far side of the dam, a unique switchback trail slices into the side of the dam and takes you to the base where you rejoin the river.

From the base of the dam, it's another 3.5 miles to the trail's terminus. The path here opens up and is once again suitable for bicyclists and equestrians. Shaded by a canopy of dense hardwood trees, you'll trace the banks of the West River to the trailhead at Jamaica State Park.

DIRECTIONS

To access the South Londonderry trailhead, take State Route 100 into the town of South Londonderry. Turn south on North River Street, and follow it to the trailhead at the road's end. (Note: Don't be deterred by private property signs along the way—keep going to the road's end.)

To reach the Jamaica State Park trailhead from South Londonderry, take State Route 100 into Jamaica, turn left onto Depot Road. Follow Depot Road to the entrance of the state park.

Contact: Friends of the West River Trail
PO Box 2086
South Londonderry, VT 05155
(802) 297-4139
www.westrivertrail.org

STAFF PICKS

Popular Rail-Trails

When Rails-to-Trails Conservancy staff members scoured New England for great rail-trails, these were the ones that stood out as their favorites. Short or long, city or country, these are rail-trails not to miss.

Connecticut
Farmington Canal Heritage Trail
Hop River State Park Trail
Middlebury Greenway

Maine
Aroostook Valley Trail
Bangor–Aroostook Trail
Eastern Promenade Trail
Narrow Gauge Pathway
Saint John Valley Heritage Trail
Whistle Stop Rail-Trail

Massachusetts
Ashuwillticook Rail Trail
Cape Cod Rail Trail
Minuteman Bikeway
Norwottuck Rail Trail

Shining Sea Bikeway
Southwest Corridor Park

New Hampshire
Cotton Valley Rail-Trail
Northern Rail-Trail – Grafton County
Rockingham Recreational Trail
Sugar River Trail

Rhode Island
Blackstone River Bikeway
East Bay Bicycle Path

Vermont
Island Line Trail
Missisquoi Valley Rail-Trail

For History Buffs

These rail-trails don't just challenge your body, they engage your mind. Pick up some historical facts on these trails.

Connecticut
Air Line State Park Trail – South

Maine
Kennebec River Rail-Trail
Saint John Valley Heritage Trail

Massachusetts
Amesbury Riverwalk
Minuteman Bikeway
Reformatory Branch Trail

New Hampshire
Cotton Valley Rail-Trail
Sugar River Trail

Rhode Island
Blackstone River Bikeway

Vermont
Toonerville Trail

40 MORE RAIL-TRAILS

There are other New England rail-trails you can investigate besides the 60 featured in this guide. The following are either very short or relatively rough and undeveloped, but like all rail-trails—they have something to offer. For more information on these additional trails, visit www.railstotrails.org to use Rails-to-Trails Conservancy's online trail-finder, TrailLink.com.

Connecticut
Air Line State Park Trail – North
Branford Trolley Trail
Railroad Ramble
Ridgefield Rail Trail
River Mills Heritage Trail
  (Putnam River Trail)

Maine
Auburn Riverwalk
Eastern Trail
Old Narrow Gauge Volunteer
  Nature Trail

Massachusetts
Blackstone River Bikeway
Connecticut Riverwalk and Bikeway
Massachusetts Central Rail Trail
  – West Boylston Section
Neponset River Trail
Old Colony Rail Trail
Quarries Footpath
Salisbury Point Ghost Train Trail
Southern New England
  Trunkline Trail
Ware River Rail Trail
WWII Veterans Memorial Trail

New Hampshire
Ammonoosuc Recreational Trail
  (Littleton to Woodsville)

Cheshire Rail Trail (Cheshire Branch
  Rail-Trail)
Dry River Trail
Fort Hill Rail-Trail
Franconia Brook Trail
Fremont Branch Rail-Trail
Granite Town Rail-Trail
Hillsborough Branch Rail-Trail
Industrial Heritage Trail
Mason Railroad Trail
Monadnock Branch Rail-Trail
Nashua Heritage Rail-Trail
Northern Rail Trail – Merrimack
  County
Presidential Range Trail
Queen City Trail
Winnipesaukee River Trail

Rhode Island
Phenix-Harris Riverwalk

Vermont
Alburg Recreational Rail-Trail
Beebe Spur
East Branch Trail
Lye Brook Trail
Montpelier & Wells River Trail (part
  of Cross Vermont Trail)

ACKNOWLEDGMENTS

Each of the trails in *Rail-Trails: New England* was personally visited by Rails-to-Trails Conservancy staff. Maps, photos, and trail descriptions are as accurate as possible thanks to the work for the following contributors:

Annalise Arkkinen

Ben Carter

Betsy Goodrich

Billy Fields

Carl Knoch

Elton Clark

Frederick Schaedtler

Gene Olig

Heather Deutsch

Jessica Leas

Kevin Hartzell

Pat Tomes

Shannon Simms

Stella Lansing

Susan Weaver

Tom Sexton

Thanks to the following for their photos:

Boyd Loving: pages vii and 159

Ryan O'Bryan: pages viii and 165

Andrea Freeman: page 129

Rails-to-Trails Conservancy would like to give special thanks to the Tawani Foundation for its generous support that helped make this guidebook possible.

tawanifoundation
distinction through transformation

INDEX

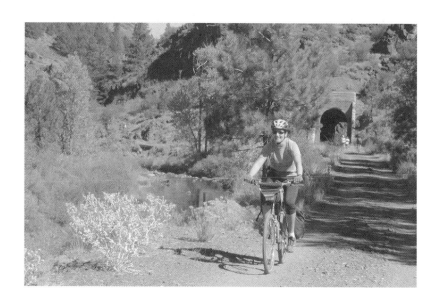

Become a member
of Rails-to-Trails Conservancy

As the nation's leader in helping communities transform unused railroad corridor into multi-use trails, Rails-to-Trails Conservancy (RTC) depends on the support of its members and donors to create access to healthy outdoor experiences.

You can help secure the future of rail-trails and enhance America's communities and countryside by becoming a member of Rails-to-Trails Conservancy today. Your donations will help support programs, projects and services that have helped put more than 13,000 rail-trail miles on the ground.

Every day, RTC provides vital technical assistance to communities throughout the country, advocates for trail-friendly policies at the local, state and national level, promotes the benefits of rail-trails and defends rail-trail laws in the courts.

Join RTC in *"inspiring movement"* and receive the following benefits:

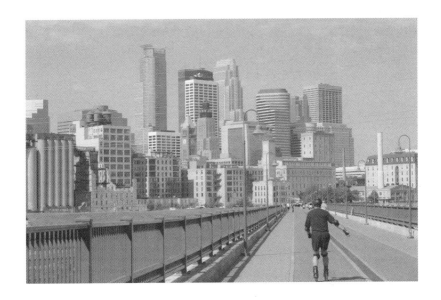

❶ New member welcome materials including *Destination Rail-Trails*, a sampler of some of the nation's finest trails

❷ A **subscription** to RTC's quarterly magazine, *Rails to Trails*.

❸ **Discounts** on publications, apparel and other merchandise including RTC's popular rail-trail guidebooks.

❹ The **satisfaction** of knowing that your dollars are helping to create a nationwide network of trails.

Membership benefits start at just $18, but additional contributions are gladly accepted.

Join online at **www.railstotrails.org**

Join by mail by sending your contribution to Rails-to-Trails Conservancy, Attention: Membership, 1100 17th St. NW, 10th Floor, Washington, DC 20036.

Join by phone by calling 1-866-202-9788.

Contributions to Rails-to-Trails Conservancy are tax deductible to the full extent of the law.

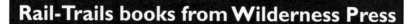